For Ian, Matthew and Jonathan

Diabetes in Hospital

A Practical Approach for Healthcare Professionals

Paula Holt

⟨W⟩WILEY-BLACKWELL

A John Wiley & Sons, Ltd., Publication

This edition first published 2009
© 2009 John Wiley & Sons, Ltd

Wiley-Blackwell is an imprint of John Wiley & Sons, formed by the merger of Wiley's global
Scientific, Technical and Medical business with Blackwell Publishing.

Registered office
John Wiley & Sons Ltd, The Atrium, Southern Gate, Chichester, West Sussex, PO19 8SQ, United
Kingdom

Editorial office
John Wiley & Sons Ltd, The Atrium, Southern Gate, Chichester, West Sussex, PO19 8SQ, United
Kingdom

For details of our global editorial offices, for customer services and for information about how to
apply for permission to reuse the copyright material in this book please see our website at
www.wiley.com/wiley-blackwell.

Library of Congress Cataloging-in-Publication Data

Holt, Paula, 1963–
    Diabetes in hospital : a practical approach for healthcare professionals / Paula Holt.
        p. ; cm.
    Includes bibliographical references and index.
    ISBN 978-0-470-72354-8 (pbk. : alk. paper)   1. Diabetes–Patients–Hospital care.   I. Title.
    [DNLM: 1. Diabetes Mellitus–therapy.   2. Hospitalization.   WK 815 H758d 2009]
    RC660.7.H65 2009
    616.4′6206–dc22
                                            2008041816

A catalogue record for this book is available from the British Library.

Set in 10/12pt Sabon by SNP Best-set Typesetter Ltd, Hong Kong
Printed in Singapore by Fabulous Printers Pte Ltd

1   2009

Contents

Preface

Today people are busier than ever but have more sedentary lifestyles. This, coupled with the increased abundance and availability of convenience foods, is contributing to rocketing levels of obesity. With this comes increasing numbers of people developing type 2 diabetes. As type 1 and type 2 diabetes transcend almost every system in the body, this will have a huge impact on health service delivery and will undoubtedly lead to more diabetes-related hospital admissions.

The aim of this book is to provide healthcare professionals with the knowledge and skills to be able to care effectively for these people during their time as a hospital in-patient. It considers the different types of specialist area a person with complications of diabetes may be admitted to, and goes on to discuss the care relevant to that person in that particular specialist setting.

The application of theory to practice is achieved through the use of different case studies to which an evidence-based, problem-solving approach is applied. The need for 'joined up', multidisciplinary working while considering fully the bio-psycho-social needs of the patient is emphasized.

The contents of the book are not 'profession specific' and readily relate to all members of the multidisciplinary team who are responsible for the care of the person with diabetes. It is aimed at providing help and guidance to those who do not have specialist knowledge of diabetes but believe their care of patients with diabetes could be improved. The advice and guidance offered is presented in a clear and logical way with evidence-based rationales so that the healthcare practitioner understands *why* they should be delivering the care in such a way.

While is it recognized that there will be an overlap of care in different care settings, the main complication for that specialism is dealt with in the appropriate chapter.

The first two chapters of the book provide the reader with the conceptual hooks that are required to understand the principles of diabetes, maintaining and achieving blood glucose control and the effective treatment of diabetes. From this, subsequent chapters focus on caring for the person with diabetes in different hospital settings and specialisms. Within each chapter, different aspects of diabetes care and complications are highlighted. Thus, the reader is able to 'dip in and out' of the chapters relating to their specialism, but if the book is read as a whole a complete picture of diabetes care is provided.

Evidence-based rationales for care are provided, drawing upon key research findings, National Institute for Health and Clinical Excellence (NICE) guidelines and the diabetes National Service Framework (NSF). A practical and logical approach is adopted with key points highlighted in boxes throughout, and at the end of each chapter. Diagrams are used to help illustrate key points.

Paula Holt
August 2008

Acknowledgements

In compiling this book I acknowledge and thank a number of people for their help, support and encouragement:

Alison Ketchell for her help with the cardiovascular implications related to diabetes and our in-depth discussions in the office about the underlying pathophysiology.

Mark Bevan and Diane Butler for their clear explanations, practical advice and support on the complexities of diabetic nephropathy and renal dialysis.

Michelle Clayton for helping me understand the role of the liver and working with me to produce articles focusing on new-onset diabetes after transplantation and hereditary haemochromatosis. The knowledge gained from these, and our discussions over coffee, have been invaluable for the book.

Janet Carling and Laura Dinning for their unconditional friendship; for facilitating clinical practice for me; and for enabling me to manage and deliver patient care, from which I have learnt a great deal.

All the people with diabetes with whom I have come into contact, including my dad, who have enriched my knowledge of diabetes and have provided me with some challenging situations to problem-solve and learn from.

Finally, my students at all academic levels, who bring to the classroom an array of experiences and clinical situations that have been drawn upon in writing this book.

Abbreviations

ABPI	Association of the British Pharmaceutical Industry
ACE	angiotensin-converting enzyme
ACEI	angiotensin-converting enzyme inhibitor
ACTH	adrenocorticotrophic hormone
ARB	angiotensin II receptor blocker
ATP	adenosine triphosphate
BMI	body mass index
DAFNE	Dose Adjustment For Normal Eating
DCCT	Diabetes Control and Complications Trial
DESMOND	Diabetes Education and Self-management for Ongoing and Newly diagnosed
DPP	Diabetes Prevention Programme
DIGAMI	Diabetes Mellitus Insulin Glucose Infusion in Acute Myocardial Infarction
DKA	diabetic ketoacidosis
DPP-4	dipeptidyl peptidase-4
DSP	distal symmetrical sensory polyneuropathy
DVLA	Driver Vehicle Licensing Agency
FREMS	frequency-modulated electromagnetic neural stimulation
GAD	glutamate decarboxylase
GFR	glomerular filtration rate
GI	glycaemic index
GIK	glucose, insulin, potassium
GIP	glucose-dependent insulinotropic polypeptide
GLP-1	glucagon-like peptide-1
GP	general practitioner
3HB	3-beta-hydroxybyturate
HbA1c	haemoglobin A1c

HDL	high-density lipoprotein
HF	high-frequency external muscle stimulation
HH	hereditary haemochromatosis
HONK	hyperosmolar, non-ketotic acidosis
HT	hyperspectral technology
IDDM	insulin-dependent diabetes mellitus
IDF	International Diabetes Federation
IDL	intermediate-density lipoprotein
IL-6	interleukin-6
LADA	latent autoimmune diabetes in adults
LDL	low-density lipoprotein
LGV	larger goods vehicles
NHS	National Health Service
NIDDM	non-insulin-dependent diabetes mellitus
MI	myocardial infarction
NAFLD	non-alcoholic fatty liver disease
NASH	non-alcoholic steatohepatitis
NEFAs	non-esterified fatty acids
NICE	National Institute for Health and Clinical Excellence
NODAT	new-onset diabetes following liver transplantation
NSF	National Service Framework
OGTT	oral glucose tolerance test
PCV	passenger-carrying vehicle
PP	pancreatic polypeptide
RAS	renin–angiotensin system
TENS	transcutaneous electrical nerve stimulation
TNFα	tumour necrosis factor α
TZDs	thiazolidinediones
UKPDS	United Kingdom Prospective Diabetes Study
VLDL	very-low-density lipoprotein
WHO	World Health Organization

1

Understanding diabetes

Aims of the chapter

This chapter will:

1. Outline the history of diabetes and insulin.
2. Identify the anatomy of the pancreas and the physiology of insulin secretion and action in a person who does not have diabetes.
3. Discuss the changes in the anatomy and physiology of insulin secretion that result in the development of both type 1 and type 2 diabetes.
4. Consider how diabetes is currently classified.
5. Discuss the aetiology and predisposing factors of type 1 and type 2 diabetes.

What is diabetes?

Diabetes mellitus is a metabolic disorder that has multiple causes and is character-ized by the continued presence of fasting plasma glucose levels >7 mmol/l, with associated disturbances of carbohydrate, fat and protein metabolism. It results from: (1) defects in insulin secretion caused by autoimmune destruction of the pancreatic beta cells; (2) insulin action due to insulin resistance; or (3) both. Insulin resistance is where the action of insulin on its target cells, namely the liver, muscle and adipose tissue, is deficient due to abnormalities of carbohydrate, fat and protein metabolism.

Diabetes is a complicated, serious, potentially debilitating and life-threatening condition, which if left uncontrolled can lead to the progressive development of a series of complications. These include: retinopathy leading to blindness; nephrop-athy that may lead to renal failure; and/or neuropathy that may result in the person having an increased risk of developing foot ulcers, limb amputation, and autonomic and sexual dysfunction. People with diabetes are also at an increased risk of developing cardiovascular disease, peripheral vascular disease and of having a cerebrovascular accident.

Diabetes currently affects 3.54% of the UK population and a known 2.2 million people in the UK have been diagnosed with the condition (Diabetes UK 2006a). However, due to the insidious nature of diabetes mellitus, Diabetes UK estimates that there are a further 750 000 to 1 million people in the UK who have diabetes, but have not yet been diagnosed. Current sedentary lifestyles and rising levels of obesity mean that the incidence of diabetes is escalating; consequently, increasing numbers of people with diabetes will be admitted to hospital with either a diabetes-related complication or their diabetes may impact on a different, non-related condition.

In order to deliver appropriate healthcare and management to the person with diabetes, it is important that the health practitioner and his or her team have an understanding of the anatomy, physiology and mechanics of diabetes and blood glucose management. The level of understanding presented in this chapter provides the groundwork upon which the remaining chapters are built.

History of diabetes and insulin

Diabetes has been recognized as a disease since ancient times – the word 'diabetes' coming from the Greek meaning 'to pass through'. It was first used by Aretaeus of Cappadocia in the 2nd century AD who described a serious condition involving the 'melting down of flesh and limbs into urine'. He went on to observe that 'life was short, unpleasant and painful, thirst unquenchable, drinking excessive and disproportionate to the large quantity of urine' (Williams and Pickup 2004). However, it was not until 1889 that diabetes began to gain significant interest from scientists and medical professionals when two German scientists, Oskar Minkowski (1858–1931) and Josef von Mering (1849–1908), discovered that when they removed the pancreas from a dog, it developed diabetes (Williams and Pickup 2004). They learnt from this that diabetes is related to a pancreatic disorder but unfortunately they did not follow up this finding.

The next major milestone in the history of diabetes came in 1921 with the discovery of insulin at the University of Toronto, Canada. Collaborative work between the surgeon Frederick G. Banting (1881–1941), one of his students Charles H. Best (1892–1965), James B. Collip (1892–1965) a biochemist, and the physiologist J.J.R. Macleod (1876–1935) found that chilling the extracts of dog pancreas and then injecting them into a dog with diabetes caused a decline in the dog's blood glucose level (Williams and Pickup 2004). From this discovery, Collip went on to develop improved procedures for the extraction and purification of insulin from pancreas, and on 1 January 1922 the first person with diabetes was treated with insulin – a 14-year-old boy called Leonard Thompson.

Based on this discovery and the experiences of Leonard Thompson, the chemists Eli Lilly and Co. from the USA jumped on to the commercial bandwagon.

They worked out processes to refine insulin extraction and purification, resulting in insulin becoming commercially available in North America and Europe from 1923. This was to have a huge impact on the treatment of people with diabetes as, up until this time, if a person developed diabetes they died due to the lack of appropriate treatment. Fortunately though, the incidence of diabetes was quite low at this time, which helped to keep the death rate low.

The past 75 years has seen the development, redevelopment and marketing of different types of insulin, with varying peak onset and action times. The supply of insulin from cow and pig pancreas is declining, resulting in the advent of new genetically modified analogue insulins introduced into the market in 1983, again by Eli Lilly. These new-generation insulins such as Humalog® and more recently Novorapid® (Novo Nordisk Ltd) have been produced via scientific technology that enables human insulin to be commercially produced from the *Escherichia coli* bacteria using recombinant DNA or cloning (Wikipedia, 2007).

This brings us right up to date with the development of inhaled insulin (Exubera®), which was prescribed to patients who met National Institute for Health and Clinical Excellence guidelines on the use of inhaled insulin (NICE 2006). Unfortunately, Exhubera® has now been withdrawn from the market as it did not meet customer's needs or financial expectations. Patients who had been prescribed the inhaled insulin have been transferred on to a different insulin regimen, but it is hoped that as the technology has now been developed Exhubera® may return to the market in the future.

Anatomy and physiology in the absence of diabetes

As can be seen from the above history, the pancreas, a major organ in the body, has a significant role to play in the normal homeostasis of blood glucose control. The pancreas is a slender, tadpole-shaped organ, pale in colour, with an uneven, lumpy consistency that sits neatly within the 'J'-shaped loop of the duodenum, deep within the greater curvature of the stomach, within the abdominal cavity. The pancreas of an adult is approximately 20–25 cm long and weighs 80 g (Martini 2006).

The pancreas has both an exocrine and an endocrine function. The exocrine pancreas, representing approximately 99% of the total pancreatic mass, is made up of pancreatic acini, which are clusters of secretory gland cells attached to ducts. The role of the glands and the associated duct cells is to secrete pancreatic digestive enzymes that drain from the pancreas via the centrally located main pancreatic duct. These digestive enzymes are required to aid the process of food digestion and absorption in the small intestine. Any trauma or condition that impairs the secretion or drainage of pancreatic digestive enzymes will seriously impair the body's ability to digest food and absorb nutrients.

The exocrine function of the pancreas does not have significant importance in diabetes. It is only the endocrine function of the pancreas that healthcare professionals involved with people who have diabetes need to be conversant with.

The endocrine pancreas consists of small clusters of cells scattered among the exocrine cells, predominantly in the body and tail of the pancreas. These clusters of cells are known as pancreatic islets or the Islets of Langerhans, named after the German anatomist Paul Langerhans in 1869. There are approximately 1 million pancreatic islet cells in the adult pancreas and each islet contains in the region of 1000 endocrine cells (Rorsman 2005).

Knowing that there are very few, if any, Islets of Langerhans in the head and neck areas of the pancreas is important, particularly if a person develops carcinoma of the head of pancreas, a tumour of the bile duct, or has acute or chronic pancreatitis. Each of these conditions may result in the person undergoing a pancreaticoduodenectomy, also known as the Whipple procedure, in which the head of the pancreas is removed. As the body and tail of the pancreas will be left, along with the alpha and beta cells, the person should not develop diabetes as a result of the surgical procedure.

Within each Islet of Langerhans there are four main types of cells, each associated with secretion of a different peptide hormone:

* Alpha (α) cells – make up approximately 20% of all cells in each Islet of Langerhans. They are predominantly situated around the periphery of the islet and secrete glucagon.
* Beta (β) cells – are the majority of the cells found in each Islet of Langerhans, accounting for 75% of the islet cells. Their function is to produce insulin.
* Delta (δ) cells – are the majority of the remaining cells in each Islet of Langerhans. These cells secrete somatostatin, which is a growth-hormone-inhibiting hormone, the effect of which is to suppress the release of glucagon and insulin and slow the rate at which food is absorbed.
* F cells – also known as PP cells as they produce the hormone pancreatic polypeptide (PP). There are very few F cells scattered throughout each Islet of Langerhans and the pancreatic polypeptide that they secrete inhibits contractions of the gallbladder and also regulates the production of some pancreatic enzymes (Martini 2006).

As the hormones insulin and glucagon are predominantly responsible for the homeostatic regulation of blood glucose levels, these will be considered in greater depth.

Insulin

Insulin is a polypeptide hormone that has a key role in the instigation of food metabolism. It is synthesized and stored in the beta cells and is released in response to the blood glucose level rising above the normal range of 4–7 mmol/l. In a healthy, normal-weight person, the average daily secretion of insulin is equivalent to 30–40 units. This is secreted via a pulsing action of the pancreas activated 300–400 times per day. It is this pulsing action, in which small amounts of insulin can be secreted frequently throughout the day and night, that makes it

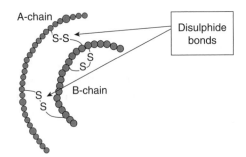

Figure 1.1   Structure of insulin.

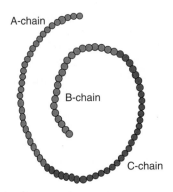

Figure 1.2   Structure of pro-insulin.

very difficult for scientists and researchers to be able to mimic the action of the pancreas accurately when giving synthetic, subcutaneous insulin. Even insulin delivered by a specially designed insulin pump, which is able to deliver insulin much more frequently than a person having insulin injections, still does not come close to the natural action of the pancreas.

Insulin consists of two polypeptide chains – an A chain of 21 residues and a B chain of 30 residues, which are joined together by two disulphide bonds (Figure 1.1).

The formation of insulin is controlled by a gene on the short arm of chromosome 11 and insulin production begins in the rough endoplasmic reticulum of the beta cells. This results in the production of pre-proinsulin, which is a precursor molecule to insulin. Pre-proinsulin is a single, long polypeptide chain containing the A chain, B chain and an additional C chain. As the development of insulin progresses, pre-proinsulin passes from the rough endoplasmic reticulum to the Golgi apparatus, still in the beta cell. During this phase it loses a chain of 24 amino acids from the end of the long chain and pro-insulin is formed (Figure 1.2). Pro-insulin has the disulphide bonds of insulin but has only one single chain of

81–86 amino acids, depending on the species, as opposed to the two separate chains of insulin (Brook and Marshall 2001). At this stage of synthesis, pro-insulin has very minimal insulin-like activity.

The C chain, also known as C-peptide, is referred to as a connecting chain as it connects the A and B chain of insulin together. C-peptide has no known biological activity but is secreted into the blood stream in equal quantities to insulin (Kettyle and Arky 1998). Occasionally, in diagnosing diabetes, the levels of C-peptide in a person's blood stream will be measured to give an indication of how much insulin, if any, the person is producing.

Within the Golgi apparatus of the beta cell, pro-insulin is converted into 'active' insulin by the cleavage of the C-peptide. When blood glucose levels begin to rise, this stimulates the need for insulin to be released and causes the A and B chains and the free floating C chain to fuse with the surface membrane of the beta cells and eventually for insulin to be released into the blood stream. The effect of this is to lower the rising blood glucose levels. Insulin can be stored in the beta cells for several days prior to its release into the blood stream. It is released into the portal vein, resulting in the liver being the first organ to be exposed to, and react to, the newly released insulin (Rorsman 2005).

Triggers for insulin secretion

As mentioned above, insulin secretion is triggered by a rising blood glucose level, which is detected in the beta cells. Conversely, insulin secretion is suppressed by falling or low blood glucose levels. The beta cells have the ability not only to detect rising or falling blood glucose levels but also to determine the rate of change in the blood glucose concentration. The beta cells are able to respond to these changes by releasing insulin at a continuous, low rate of approximately 1–2 units per hour. This is called the 'basal rate' or late-phase insulin release. Yet the beta cells are also able to secrete insulin at much higher levels for a short period of time in response to a rapidly rising blood glucose level which happens, for example, just after the person has eaten. This is known as a 'bolus' or early-phase insulin release and will have implications when insulin treatments are discussed in Chapter 2.

There are three main situations in which insulin release will be triggered:

- An increase in blood glucose concentrations.
- An increase in amino acid concentrations.
- Increased parasympathetic input.

1. Increase in blood glucose concentrations

When both simple and complex carbohydrate foods such as pasta, potatoes, bread, cakes, sweets, etc. are eaten, the sugar from these foods gets absorbed from the stomach and small intestine into the blood stream, causing a rise in blood glucose concentrations.

2. Increase in amino acid concentrations

Amino acids are fundamental constituents of protein and can be found in the protein in our diet, as well as being synthesized by the body. Between meals or during a fast, amino acids are released from muscle cells into the blood stream. When they reach the liver, in response to a falling blood glucose level, the liver converts the amino acids into glucose via a process called gluconeogenesis. This 'new' glucose is then transported into the blood stream and blood glucose levels rise. At the same time the glucose that has been stored in the liver in the form of glycogen is broken down by a process known as glycogenolysis, meaning the breakdown of glycogen, and again released into the blood stream. These processes are part of the body's compensatory mechanism to ensure that the vital organs such as kidneys and brain, which do not have insulin receptors, obtain their continuous required levels of glucose.

3. Increased parasympathetic output

As part of the 'fight or flight' sympathetic mechanism, which is triggered when faced with a dangerous, difficult or frightening situation, the body will make and release glucose to provide the person with the extra energy that may be required to escape the situation. This results in blood glucose levels becoming raised. Once the fight or flight situation has abated, the parasympathetic nervous system triggers the release of insulin to reduce the elevated blood glucose levels back to within normal limits.

Effects of insulin on target cells

The mechanisms by which insulin reduces blood glucose levels are now considered. The main aim of this process is to remove the circulating glucose from the blood steam either by utilizing it for energy and growth, absorbing and storing it elsewhere in the form of glycogen, or converting it into triglycerides. This is achieved via a number of different mechanisms (Figure 1.3).

Insulin degradation

Once secreted, insulin is rapidly degraded and removed from the circulation by the liver and kidneys. This is done by breaking down the disulphide bonds that connect the A and B chain together. This occurs quite rapidly after secretion, giving insulin an active biological half-life of only 6–10 minutes. It is expected that all insulin produced will be broken down within 12–20 minutes of it being secreted, which highlights the need for the pancreas to produce insulin on average 300–400 times per day. This biologically short life of insulin helps to ensure that the ever-fluctuating blood glucose levels are kept within the normal range of 4–7 mmol/l and the person does not experience frequent hypoglycaemic episodes.

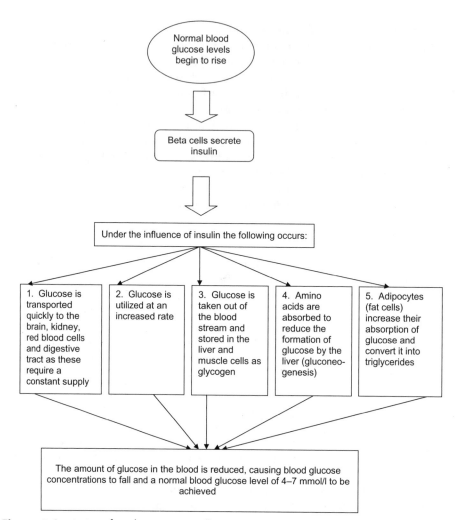

Figure 1.3 Action of insulin on target cells.

Glucagon

Glucagon, which is secreted by the alpha cells in the Islets of Langerhans, has an equal part to play with insulin in the regulation of blood glucose levels. While the action of insulin causes blood glucose levels to fall, glucagon has the opposite effect and causes them to rise. Similarly, the release of glucagon is stimulated by falling blood glucose levels and suppressed by the release of insulin, which is secreted when blood glucose levels rise.

When blood glucose levels start to fall, the sequence of events shown in Figure 1.3 is reversed. The body mobilizes its stores of glycogen that have been laid down under the influence of insulin in the liver and muscle cells. By converting glycogen back to glucose through the process of glycogenolysis, this enables glucose to be either metabolized for energy or absorbed back into the blood stream, resulting in an increase in blood glucose levels.

At the same time, falling blood glucose levels stimulate the liver to absorb amino acids from the blood stream and convert them to glucose by the process of gluconeogenesis; this 'manufactured' glucose is then released into the blood stream to increase blood glucose levels.

In addition to this, the triglycerides that were converted from glucose and stored in the adipocytes are broken down into fatty acids and transported around the body via the circulatory system, to be utilized by other tissues. Each of these pathways combines, with the ultimate aim of increasing blood glucose levels to prevent hypoglycaemia.

Interestingly, glucagon is also secreted in response to an increase in plasma amino acid concentration, which is contradictory to the process mentioned earlier. An increase in plasma amino acid concentration also stimulates the release of the conflicting hormone insulin. This is a safety mechanism to prevent the occurrence of hypoglycaemia, with would threaten the fuel supply to the brain.

If a person eats a meal that is high in protein and does not contain any carbo-hydrates, the body will respond to this by secreting insulin to reduce the plasma amino acid concentration. As the meal did not contain carbohydrates, the person's blood glucose level will not rise significantly, yet insulin is being secreted thus lowering the blood glucose level and potentially causing hypoglycaemia. Some-thing needs to counteract this process and this is achieved by the release of glu-cagon by liver and muscle cells. While in this situation, insulin and glucagon are being secreted together and the body will respond to the hormone that is most prevalent in the blood stream at a given time. In this case, glucagon will be secreted to prevent blood glucose levels falling.

Classification of diabetes

Over the years diabetes has been classified in many different ways and people with diabetes have been given a variety of labels. In the early 1970s, age was used to classify diabetes and people were described as having 'juvenile-onset' or 'mature-onset' diabetes. In the 1980s, diabetes was largely categorized by the type of treat-ment a person received for their diabetes, leading to them being labelled as having insulin-dependent diabetes mellitus (IDDM) or non-insulin-dependent diabetes mellitus (NIDDM). These terms were not particularly flattering, but the course of diabetes generally meant that there was a propensity for juveniles or young people approaching and entering teenage years to develop diabetes and it was this group of people that would be need to be commenced on subcutaneous insulin therapy from the time of diagnosis. They would then be labelled a 'juvenile-onset IDDM'.

If a person was lucky enough to escape diabetes by the end of their teens, a diagnosis was rarely made in middle-aged people and the incidence tended to peak again with old age, 60 years and over, hence the term 'mature-onset'. In this group of people the focus of treatment was to modify diet and exercise. If this was not successful, the person would commence on a sulphonylurea drug such as chlorpropamide or glibenclamide to enhance beta-cell production of insulin. It was unusual for these people to commence on insulin as the stringent blood glucose targets that we have in place today did not apply 20 years ago, and the person with diabetes generally died before insulin was required as a treatment option.

In 1980, the World Health Organization published the first widely accepted classification of diabetes (WHO 1980). It was then decided, based on the literature at the time, that there should be two major classes of diabetes mellitus – IDDM or type 1 and NIDDM or type 2. However, in 1985 the terms type 1 and type 2 were omitted leaving just IDDM and NIDDM as the main classifications. These terms were generally accepted and used internationally (WHO, 1999).

In the early 1990s, knowledge was beginning to emerge regarding the aetiology and pathogenesis of diabetes, which led many eminent individuals and groups of people in the field of diabetes to question whether the classification needed to be altered again. Diabetes was changing – no longer were patients with IDDM being diagnosed as teenagers, but people in their 30s and 40s were also developing diabetes that needed to be controlled by insulin from the outset. In addition, those who had traditionally been labelled as NIDDM were now beginning to commence insulin therapy as a means of reducing their blood glucose levels in order to meet the healthcare targets for blood glucose levels. The role of obesity and lifestyle in diabetes was also becoming more apparent and researchers were questioning whether juvenile-onset diabetes and mature-onset diabetes were actually two different, but similar, conditions.

Concerns were raised in the medical professions about having a medical labelling system that classifies such a potentially serious condition on the type of pharmacological treatment used to manage the condition. This type of classification was also found to be confusing – NIDDM patients were changing their classification once they commenced on insulin, which was not helpful in understanding the person's diabetes. Calls were made to have a classification based, where possible, on the disease aetiology (American Diabetes Association 2003).

For these reasons an International Expert Committee was set up in 1995, working under the support of the American Diabetes Association, to review the scientific literature that had been published since the last classification in 1980 and decide if changes to the classification of diabetes were warranted (American Diabetes Association 2003). In 1999, the International Expert Committee proposed that the terms IDDM and NIDDM be eliminated. Instead, diabetes should be classified as type 1 and type 2 with the use of Arabic numerals instead of Roman numerals to prevent the public from confusing II with the number 11 (American Diabetes Association 2003). Therefore, the only terms that should be used in clinical practice today to determine types of diabetes are type 1 or type 2.

> **Key point**
>
> The only terms that should be used to determine the type of diabetes a person has are type 1 and type 2.

As is explained below, type 1 and type 2 diabetes are essentially quite different conditions but both affect the overall control of blood glucose levels. It is important to recognize and understand the differences between the two conditions. In particular, it is important to understand that a person who is accurately diagnosed as having type 2 diabetes does *not* become a person with type 1 diabetes once they commence insulin therapy. This appears to be a common misconception in clinical practice and the reasons why this does, and should, not happen will become clear with the following explanations of the different types of diabetes.

> **Key point**
>
> A person with type 2 diabetes who then commences insulin therapy does *not* become a person with type 1 diabetes. They are a person with type 2 diabetes requiring insulin therapy.

Type 1 diabetes

Type 1 diabetes is a chronic autoimmune disease in which the T lymphocytes infiltrate the insulin-producing beta cells of the pancreas and progressively destroy them (Faideau 2005), resulting in the production of little or no insulin (Pozzilli and Mario 2001). The rate of beta-cell destruction varies quite considerably between individuals. There is a tendency for it to be quite rapid in infants and children, and slower in adults (Zimmet *et al.* 1994). By the time a person begins to develop the signs and symptoms of type 1 diabetes, over 90% of their beta cells will have been destroyed; this causes a marked insulin deficiency, which is the hallmark of type 1 diabetes.

Immune-mediated diabetes typically occurs in childhood and adolescence but it is important to remember that it can occur at any age. Even someone in their 8th or 9th decade can develop type 1 diabetes and it should therefore not be ruled out (American Diabetes Association 2003).

Predisposing factors

A common characteristic of people who develop type 1 diabetes is that they are predominantly young and thin. However, this is not to say that older and heavier people do not develop type 1 diabetes, it is just that it tends to be less common in this group.

Approximately 10–15% of the total population of people who have diabetes will have type 1 diabetes, and there is not doubt that young-onset type 1 diabetes is increasing in frequency in most western countries, particularly in children younger than 5 years (Bonifacio *et al.* 2004).

Familial/genetic link

There is convincing evidence that type 1 diabetes runs in families. Bonifacio *et al.* (2004) found that, depending on which family member had diabetes, the offspring's probability of developing type 1 diabetes was increased or decreased by the age of 5 years (Table 1.1).

Bonifacio *et al.* (2004) also looked at the risk of children with a family history of developing type 1 diabetes, themselves going on to develop multiple islet auto-antibodies (a strong precursor to type 1 diabetes) but not necessarily type 1 diabetes by the age of 5 years. Table 1.2 details the results of this study.

The study also questioned whether there was any difference in the potential to develop multiple islet autoantibodies if the parent was either the mother or the father. Interestingly, the risk was higher in the offspring of fathers with type 1 diabetes (4.2% by 5 years of age) compared to the offspring of mothers with type 1 diabetes (2.4% by 5 years of age). This risk was further exacerbated in children who had a parent with a first-degree family history of type 1 diabetes, compared to those who have not (Bonifacio *et al.* 2004).

The above findings clearly demonstrate a familial/genetic link in the development of type 1 diabetes but environmental factors have also been thought to play a part. A genetic predisposition to diabetes needs to be present and the strength of the link between this and the development of diabetes depends on the level of aggressiveness of the environmental factors (Akerblom *et al.* 2002).

Table 1.1 Offspring risk of developing type 1 diabetes.

Offspring who have . . .	Risk of developing type 1 diabetes by age 5 years (%)
Both parents with type 1 diabetes	10.9
A parent and a sibling with type 1 diabetes	11.8
One parent with type 1 diabetes	0.8

Table 1.2 Offspring risk of developing multiple islet autoantibodies.

Offspring who have . . .	Risk of developing multiple islet autoantibodies (%)
One parent and no sibling with type 1 diabetes	3.0
Both parents with type 1 diabetes	23.3
One parent and a sibling with type 1 diabetes	30.4

Environmental factors

In a worldwide project conducted between 1990 and 1999, it was calculated that the overall incidence of type 1 diabetes in children aged up to and including 14 years varied enormously across the globe. The incidence in China and Venezuela was 0.1 per 100000/year while in Finland the figure was 40.9 per 100000/year, demonstrating a huge variation according to location. The average annual increase calculated from 103 centres worldwide was 2.8% (DIAMOND project group 2006). While this high annual increase in incidence may be partly attributable to the improvements made in diabetes screening and reporting mechanisms, recent studies have shown that environmental factors have a significant role to play in the development of type 1 diabetes (Hermann *et al.* 2003; Kaila *et al.* 2003; Gillespie *et al.* 2004).

Numerous studies have tried, and continue to try, to explain the possible reasons why a person may progressively destroy their own beta cells. A number of researchers have suggested the potential involvement of various environmental factors.

1. Viral infections

Several studies have suggested that viral infections may have a role to play in the development of type 1 diabetes (Menser *et al.* 1978). In particular, a link was made between measles, mumps and rubella and type 1 diabetes. However, with the introduction of an effective vaccination programme over recent years, the incidence of rubella has fallen dramatically yet the incidence of type 1 diabetes continues to rise. It will be interesting to see if there is any correlation between rubella and type 1 diabetes now that parents are actively opting not to have their children vaccinated with the triple measles, mumps and rubella vaccine, as this will undoubtedly increase the incidence of these conditions in the western world.

Currently, enterovirus is being seen as a predominant viral trigger for type 1 diabetes. Enterovirus infections are prevalent among children and adolescents, corresponding with the main age of diabetes onset. The virus is predominantly found in the lymphoid tissues of the pharynx and small intestine, but as it enters the blood stream is can spread to various organs, including the pancreas (Akerblom *et al.* 2002), resulting in damage to the beta cells. This link has been made due to antigens to enterovirus being found in both children with type 1 diabetes and prediabetic children (Jones and Crosby 1996). In addition, Clements *et al.* (1995) detected enterovirus in the blood of 27–64% of patients with newly diagnosed type 1 diabetes.

2. Early exposure to cow's milk

The cows' milk and type 1 diabetes hypothesis has been considered and debated for more than 20 years. Research using mice clearly demonstrated a deleterious effect of the proteins found in cows' milk in the development of type 1 diabetes (Elliott *et al.* 1988). In addition, Norris and Scott (1996) reported that babies who were breast fed for less than 3–4 months had a two-fold risk of type 1 diabetes. However, Vaarala *et al.* (1999) reported that exposure to cows' milk proteins *per se* does not cause diabetes, rather it is the mechanisms by which our bodies tolerate these proteins that can trigger type 1 diabetes.

3. Deficiency of vitamin D
Experiments in mice have shown that supplementing their diet with an active form of vitamin D prevents both the occurrence of insulitis, which damages beta cells, and the development of autoimmune diabetes. Furthermore, the EURODIAB Substudy 2 study group (1999) reported that giving vitamin D supplements in infancy significantly decreased the risk of developing type 1 diabetes. Cod liver oil administration during pregnancy has also been found to be associated with a decreased risk of type 1 diabetes in the offspring (Stene *et al.* 2000).

4. Obesity
Evidence is also emerging that rapid growth and obesity in early childhood increases the risk of type 1 diabetes due to the increased need for insulin, which the body struggles to cope with. Obesity also plays a significant role in the development of type 2 diabetes, as will be seen later.

5. Toxins
Alloxan and streptozotocin have been found to damage beta cells at different sites, resulting in reduced insulin secretion. The rat poison Vacor has also been linked to the onset of type 1 diabetes in humans and it is thought that it has a similar action to streptozotocin. Bafilomycins, which are found in infected soil, have been shown to contaminate vegetable plant roots and tubers. As these vegetables are readily available and current dietary trends advocate a minimum of five portions of fruit and vegetables daily for maximum health, there is a ready route for bafilomycins to enter the body. Researchers believe that bafilomycins may play a role in promoting diabetes if a fetus is exposed to them *in utero*. In a study on non-obese mice with diabetes, Hettiarachchi *et al.* (2004) found that exposure to bafilomycin across the placenta disrupts the development of the fetal pancreas, which in turn predisposes to diabetes in infancy. Their study did not link the infection of bafilomycin after birth with the development of diabetes.

Type 2 diabetes

The aetiology of type 2 diabetes is quite different from type 1 and the new classification system for diabetes takes this into account.

Type 2 diabetes is predominantly linked to obesity and a sedentary lifestyle, which results in insulin resistance. Thus people who develop type 2 diabetes are often overweight and older. Approximately 75–80% of patients with type 2 diabetes have been or are obese (body mass index [BMI] >24.9 kg/m^2). Indeed, it has been shown that, on average, for every 1 kg increase in body weight a person has a 9% relative increase in the risk of developing type 2 diabetes (Mokdad *et al.* 2000). Type 2 diabetes accounts for 85–90% of the total population who have diabetes and affects approximately 3% of the population of the UK (Diabetes UK 2006a).

Traditionally, type 2 diabetes, essentially equivalent to the old 'mature-onset' diabetes, was only diagnosed in people who were classed middle to old aged. However, today there is an increased prevalence of childhood obesity; this has reached epidemic proportions in both the developed and developing world (Reilly 2004). This has serious implications on the aetiology of type 2 diabetes. Diabetes practitioners are now coming into contact with children as young as 8 years old diagnosed with type 2 diabetes. This means that the children have to live with, and control, their diabetes for much longer, putting them at much greater risk of developing diabetes-related complications that can not only seriously reduce life expectancy (Haslam and James 2005) but also increase the financial burden on an already 'cash-strapped' National Health Service in the UK.

In contrast to type 1 diabetes, type 2 diabetes is very insidious in nature. It is well documented that a person can have type 2 diabetes up to 12 years before symptoms appear and a diagnosis is made. As a consequence, 50% of people may have already developed one or more complication of diabetes at the time of diagnosis.

Insulin resistance

Up to 25% of the population in the UK is thought to have a level of insulin resistance similar to those people who have type 2 diabetes and it is known that insulin resistance predates the development of diabetes by many years, but it is not thought sufficient to cause diabetes by itself. Impaired beta cell function must also be present at the same time.

Insulin resistance predominantly affects those who are obese and 'apple-shaped', i.e. who have a low waist to hip ratio. It is the laying down of visceral, abdominal, fat that affects the efficiency of the secreted insulin and contributes to mechanisms that actively increase blood glucose levels and worsen the situation. This is achieved in three different ways:

1. Loss of insulin receptors
Insulin receptors are present in most cell membranes, except cells in the brain, kidneys, lining of the digestive tract and red blood cells. These types of cells lack insulin receptors as they have the unique ability to absorb and utilize glucose, independent of insulin. For this reason they require an adequate, regular and controlled amount of glucose in order to function appropriately.

Where present, insulin receptors are found on the surface of cells (Figure 1.4). As blood glucose levels rise and insulin is secreted, the insulin 'unlocks the door' of the insulin receptor to allow glucose and insulin to enter the cell thus reducing blood glucose levels. At this time, the insulin receptor is also internalized within the cell. Once this process is complete the insulin receptor is recycled back on the surface of the cell to begin the process again.

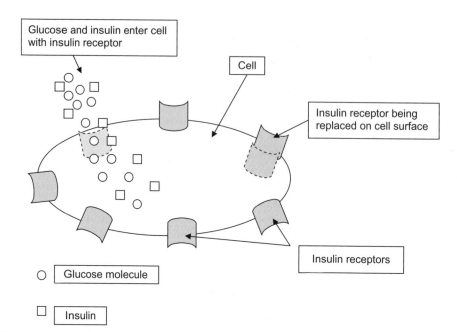

Figure 1.4 Insulin receptors and internalization of glucose and insulin.

In type 2 diabetes, over a period of time, the insulin receptors are not replaced on the surface of the cells, which means that there are less 'doors' by which glucose can enter the cells and be removed from the blood stream. This causes blood glucose levels to rise. This rise is detected by the beta cells, which respond by further increasing the secretion of insulin, thinking that this is the cause of the problem. As this is not the case, this insulin has limited effect on the blood glucose level. This state of *hyperinsulinaemia* further exacerbates the insulin resistance and pushes the beta cells to work extremely hard in producing and secreting insulin. After a while the beta cells find responding to this increased need difficult, become exhausted and die, resulting in less and less insulin being produced.

These effects of insulin resistance are also compounded by the infiltration of fat cells into the pancreatic islet cells, which also causes premature and rapid decline in the beta cells' ability to maintain an increased insulin output (Haslam and James 2005).

At this time the person usually begins to develop signs and symptoms of type 2 diabetes. Hyperinsulinaemia resulting in insulin resistance also creates other metabolic risk factors, such as raised blood pressure and hyperlipidaemia (Broom 2006), which are discussed later.

2. Distribution of fat

The central abdominal visceral fat distribution of 'apple-shaped' people also contributes to the development of type 2 diabetes. This type of fat is highly metabolically active; as it breaks down it releases large amounts of non-esterified fatty acids (NEFAs). These NEFAs act to increase gluconeogenesis (formation of new glucose) in the liver and impair the uptake and utilization of glucose in the muscle cells, leading to a deleterious rise in blood glucose levels.

3. Tumour necrosis factor

In addition, adipose tissue (fat cells) produce tumour necrosis factor α, resistin and interleukin 6 (IL-6), which are cytokines that have been shown to interfere in a negative way with the action of insulin (Williams and Pickup 2004).

As can be seen, the causes of type 1 and type 2 diabetes are not the same and, as a result, treatment will differ. These differences highlight how, once an accurate diagnosis of diabetes has been made, a person cannot cross over to the other type, regardless of the treatment they require.

Predisposing factors for type 2 diabetes

There are a number of predisposing factors that have been associated with an increased likelihood for developing type 2 diabetes. The more predisposing factors a person has, the more likely they are to develop type 2 diabetes.

1. Ethnic group

South Asian and Afro-Caribbean people are at a substantially increased risk of developing diabetes. It has been confirmed that this group of people are five times more likely to develop type 2 diabetes than white people (Diabetes UK 2006a). In addition, South Asian and Afro-Caribbean people develop diabetes around a decade earlier than their Caucasian counterparts and at a lower level of obesity. This means that they have a longer period over which to control their blood glucose levels to avoid the risks of diabetes-related complications.

Evolutionary changes have led to this high risk. These people have traditionally lived with difficult nutritional conditions and so have developed high efficiency in the metabolism of carbohydrates. This has also been helped by high levels of exercise while tending land and collecting water. However, as these ethnic groups have become increasingly 'westernized' and have adopted an increasingly sedentary lifestyle, with access to an abundance of processed, high-fat and high-sugar foods, their once highly efficient metabolism cannot cope with these changes and their beta cells are unable to produce enough insulin to control blood glucose levels. Ultimately, type 2 diabetes results.

This has been termed the 'thrifty-gene hypothesis' and it has been postulated that genes predisposing to type 2 diabetes might have been survival genes, helping people to store surplus energy as abdominal fat during periods of extreme starvation. However, when exposed to the sedentary lifestyle and high calorie intake of the modern, western world, these genes predispose to obesity, insulin resistance and, subsequently, type 2 diabetes.

2. Obesity and reduced physical activity

It is well documented that obesity and weight gain are major risk factors in the development of type 2 diabetes (Maggio and Pi-Sunyer 1997), but these risk factors have been shown to increase even when a person has a BMI as low as 21.0 kg/m^2 (James *et al.* 2005, cited in Haslam and James 2005). As has been shown, the accumulation of intra-abdominal fat as seen in apple-shaped people acts as an independent diabetogenic risk factor. People today are busier than ever and are more inclined to choose readily available, high-density, calorie- and fat-laden convenience foods over home-cooked meals made from freshly prepared ingredients. These factors are compounded by a food industry that actively promotes overeating with the marketing of 'larger' and 'supersize' portions (Cowburn 2004).

Coupled with this are the reduced levels of physical activity that are found today. Owing to advancements in technology over recent years, in both the workplace and the home, people tend to lead far more sedentary lifestyles than their predecessors, and consequently do not use the same amount of energy doing simple everyday tasks. Furthermore, the advent of computers and game stations has negatively impacted on exercise levels of children and adults. Children, especially, are now more likely to sit in front of a television or computer screen playing computer generated games rather than being outside playing activity games or riding bicycles.

Thus both lack of exercise and high-calorie diets are major contributors to rising obesity levels and subsequent insulin resistance.

3. Advancing age

All body systems become less efficient and more likely to fail as we age. Beta cells in the pancreas are no exception to this and it is accepted that there will be a decline in beta-cell mass and function as we get older. Over the age of 45 years, beta-cell function declines but the rate of decline largely depends on the workload of the beta cells, which is determined by the level and duration of insulin resistance.

4. Thrifty phenotype hypothesis

The 'thrifty phenotype hypothesis' (Hales and Barker 2001) applies to babies of low birth weight (under 2.3 kg). It is suspected from their low birth weight that the nutritional conditions in the uterus have been suboptimal, resulting in a degree of fetal malnourishment causing decreased islet-cell function and impaired beta-cell growth. In response, the fetus develops hormonal and metabolic adaptations to cope with the situation, including being nutritionally 'thrifty'. The low-birth-weight baby therefore enters adulthood with a decreased number of beta cells; if at this time nutrition is good or there is evidence of obesity, this will expose the impaired islet-cell function, which will also be exacerbated with advancing age, and type 2 diabetes will result.

5. Smoking

Cigarette smoking was first highlighted as a predisposing factor to the development of type 2 diabetes in the late 1980s. Since then, only a few prospective studies have considered the relationship between the frequency of cigarette smoking and the incidence of diabetes mellitus. Will *et al.* (2001) carried out a study to determine whether the onset of diabetes was related to the number of cigarettes a person smoked and whether quitting reversed the effect. They found that, as the number of cigarettes smoked increased, so did the rate of diabetes in both men and women. Men who smoked more than 40 cigarettes a day had a 45% higher diabetes rate than men who had never smoked; the comparable increase for women was 74%. These are obviously highly significant results and clearly demonstrate a link between smoking and the onset of diabetes. Will *et al.* (2001) also found that by stopping smoking, the rate of diabetes reduced to that of non-smokers after 5 years in women and 10 years in men.

Attempts have been made to understand the biological mechanisms underpinning these findings. Some investigators have suggested that cigarette smoking generally increases insulin resistance by altering the distribution of body fat or by exerting a direct toxin on pancreatic tissue (Rimm *et al.* 1995). Shepherd and Kahn (1999) questioned whether a chemical component of cigarettes may directly alter the transport mechanism that allows glucose to enter the cells from the blood stream, thus contributing to hyperglycaemia. This was also considered by Rincon *et al.* (1999), who found that insulin-stimulated glucose transport in the skeletal muscle of smokers was moderately impaired in comparison with non smokers. As cigarettes contain 3500 different particle compounds and 500 gaseous compounds, defining which compound is responsible for the alteration in glucose transport would be a difficult and formidable task; however, evidence certainly suggests a link between smoking and diabetes.

6. Psychological stress

The contribution of psychological stress on the development of diabetes is being investigated with increasing attention. During periods of acute or chronic stress, the sympathetic nervous system increases levels of adrenaline in the body. This has the affect of increasing blood glucose levels – the 'fight or flight' mechanism. Under normal circumstances the body is able to deal with these increased blood glucose levels by increasing the amount of insulin secreted. In someone who has a predisposition to diabetes, or who may already have diabetes but have not been formally diagnosed, the presence of psychological stress may be enough to 'tip the balance' between being able to control blood glucose levels and not being able to. People will quite often comment on what a stressful time they had been going through before they developed diabetes. However, it is not always clear which came first – the diabetes or the stress.

7. Exposure to pesticides

Recently, researchers have found that long-term exposure to pesticides increases a person's risk of developing type 2 diabetes. A study by Montgomery *et al.* (2008), which involved more than 33 000 people working with pesticides, found that exposure to seven pesticides (aldrin, chlordane, heptachlor, dichlorvos, trichlorfon, alachlor and cyanazine) increased workers' risk of developing diabetes.

It was also found that the incidence of diabetes increased with increased exposure to the pesticide.

8. Drinking fruit juice

Women who drink a glass of fruit juice each morning may be 18% more likely to develop type 2 diabetes (Bazzano *et al.* 2008). Whether the same applies to men is not known as the study by only recruited females and followed their dietary habits for 18 years. The same results were not found when the women ate the whole fruit, instead of just consuming the juice. This suggests that naturally occurring sugar in fruit causes a sharp rise in blood glucose levels as it quickly passes through the digestive system. Women with any degree of insulin resistance or beta-cell impairment will not be able to cope with this high glucose excursion on a regular basis and the onset of diabetes may result.

Signs and symptoms of diabetes

Signs and symptoms of diabetes vary considerably in their severity and rate of onset. Typically, in someone with type 1 diabetes the symptoms will develop fairly quickly, usually over a few weeks, or sometimes over just a few days. With type 2 diabetes, the symptoms can develop much more gradually – it often has a slow and insidious onset, with many cases of diabetes going undetected for years due to the lack of symptoms.

The classical signs and symptoms of increasing blood glucose levels, which occur in both type 1 and type 2 diabetes, are shown below.

Polyuria

This is the production of large amounts of dilute urine and is the body and kidney's response to rising blood glucose levels. The kidneys increase their output in an attempt to excrete the excess glucose but in doing so they also excrete large amounts of water, which causes significant dehydration. This can give rise to bed-wetting in some children and incontinence in the elderly.

Thirst

Owing to the dehydration caused by the excessive action of the kidneys to excrete glucose, the person becomes very thirsty and complains that their mouth is so dry their tongue feels as if it is sticking to the roof of their mouth. To compensate, the person drinks copious amounts of fluids, which often may contain high levels of sugar, thus worsening the condition. It is important to remember that in diabetes it is the polyuria that comes first and causes the dehydration and thirst, not the other way round.

Glycosuria

Under normal, non-diabetes circumstances, the kidneys do not allow glucose to enter the urine if the blood glucose concentration is below 8 mmol/l, but this depends on the individual's renal threshold, which can alter. Some people may not begin to excrete glucose in the urine until their blood glucose levels rise above 10 mmol/l. Once the person's renal threshold has been reached, glucose starts to leak into the urine and as it does, the syrupy urine draws water with it, causing dehydration.

Weight loss

As there is a general shortage of active insulin, either due to poor insulin secretion or insulin resistance, blood glucose is prevented from being stored in the liver, skeletal muscle cells and adipose tissue where it would normally be converted into energy when required. Thus, the body seeks energy from different sources, including the breakdown of protein from muscle; this results in weight loss, which can range from a 1–2 kg to over 50 kg in more severe cases.

Tiredness and weakness

As there are no energy stores, as explained above, the person often comments on feeling continually very tired. This symptom is often overlooked, owing to the hectic lifestyles many people lead today. Some people complain of falling asleep at odd times, while others initially put this symptom down to lifestyle and/or growing old before their time. The feeling of tiredness is often accompanied by a sensation of weakness and lethargy as glucose is unable to enter the muscle cells to give the person strength.

Blurring of vision

The high level of glucose in the body changes the osmotic pressure in the eye, which causes the lens of the eye to change slightly in shape. This can result in the person becoming acutely short-sighted or, alternatively, they may find reading very difficult. Once a diagnosis of diabetes has been made and blood glucose levels have been returned to normal, the person's sight will normally be fully restored within 2–3 weeks. It is therefore wise not to recommend that the person has an eye test for at least 1 month after proper stabilization of the diabetes has been achieved.

Skin infections and genital soreness

Bacteria on the skin thrive on the large amounts of glucose circulating in the blood stream, giving rise to recurrent boils, skin infections and genital thrush. In addition, the large quantities of glucose passed in the urine tend to create soreness around the genital area. These unpleasant problems rapidly disappear once the diabetes is controlled and the blood glucose levels return to normal.

Making a diagnosis

In making a diagnosis of diabetes, the clinician must feel confident that the diagnosis is accurate as the potential consequences for the individual are considerable and life-long.

Currently, the World Health Organization (WHO) criteria for diagnosing diabetes is used in practice. A diagnosis should only be made when the person tests positive in at least two of the following criteria: (1) presence of symptoms; (2) abnormal random venous blood glucose level; and (3) abnormal fasting venous blood glucose level. If this cannot be achieved or the venous blood glucose results are borderline, a 2-hour oral glucose tolerance test (OGTT) may be required to confirm or refute the diagnosis.

For an OGTT, the patient is required to fast from midnight on the day of the test. They will then attend a laboratory where a fasting blood glucose level will be recorded. The patient will then be asked to swallow 75 g of glucose, usually either in water or in the form of Lucozade®. A tip here is if the 75 g of glucose is being given in water, make sure that the water is given to the patient at body temperature. This allows the patient to drink the contents rapidly as the taste is very unpleasant.

Following the ingestion of the glucose, the person's blood glucose level will generally be recorded every 30 minutes up to and including 2 hours post-glucose drink. Under normal circumstances, an OGTT would not be required as it is unpleasant and costly in terms of patient and laboratory time.

Table 1.3 identifies the blood glucose values required to make a diagnosis of diabetes mellitus. It also highlights the blood glucose assay of other categories of hyperglycaemia which may indicate a propensity to develop diabetes.

Table 1.3 Values for diagnosis of diabetes mellitus and other categories of hyperglycaemia. Adapted from WHO (2006).

	Glucose concentration (mmol/l)		
	Whole blood venous	Whole blood capillary	Plasma
Diabetes mellitus			
Fasting OR	≥6.1	≥6.1	≥7.0
2 hour post 75 g glucose load (OGTT)	≥10.0	≥11.1	≥11.1
Impaired glucose tolerance			
Fasting AND	<6.1 and ≥6.7	<6.1 and ≥7.8	<7.0 and ≥7.8
2 hour post 75 g glucose load			
Impaired fasting glycaemia			
Fasting	≥5.6 and <6.1	≥5.6 and <6.1	≥6.1 and <7.0
2 hour post 75 g glucose load	<6.7	<7.8	<7.8

OGTT, oral glucose tolerance test.

In a fraction of individuals with type 1 diabetes, the rate of autoimmune beta cell destruction is very slow; as their diabetes is not initially insulin requiring they appear to be clinically affected by type 2 diabetes. These patients are clinically difficult to distinguish from type 2 diabetes subjects. The presence or absence of islet autoantibodies such as glutamate decarboxylase (GAD) is one of the more reliable ways to distinguish between type 1 and type 2 diabetes. People with type 1 diabetes will have GAD antibodies present in their blood, whereas those with type 2 will not as their diabetes is not triggered by an autoimmune response.

The term latent autoimmune diabetes in adults (LADA) has been introduced to define adult patients with diabetes who do not require insulin initially but have the immune markers of type 1 diabetes. The majority of these patients will eventually progress to insulin dependency (Pozzilli and Mario 2001).

Conclusion

Within this chapter the history of insulin discovery and diabetes dating back to the 2nd century AD has been outlined and brought up to date with the development of new analogue insulins currently on the pharmaceutical market.

The anatomy of the pancreas and the physiology of insulin secretion and action have been described and how abnormalities of this result in the development of type 1 and type 2 diabetes. Despite both being related to the secretion of insulin, it has been shown that these two conditions are quite different, with different risk factors. The historical classification of diabetes was discussed, and emphasis placed on how the classification of diabetes in relation to its treatment needed to be reviewed in order to respond to the changing face of diabetes today.

Finally, the aetiology and predisposing factors that increase a person's risk of developing type 1 or type 2 diabetes were discussed and rationales provided. Classical signs and symptoms of diabetes were outlined, along with current WHO criteria for diagnosing diabetes.

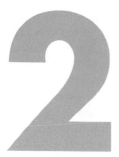

Treating diabetes effectively

Aims of the chapter

This chapter will:

1. Consider clinical situations in which insulin therapy will be required.
2. Distinguish between and discuss different insulin preparations and their uses in clinical practice.
3. Review the role of diet and lifestyle in the treatment of diabetes.
4. Consider the range of oral antidiabetes medications and their use in clinical practice.
5. Offer discussion of two case study scenarios related to the pharmacological treatment of diabetes.

The aetiology and incidence of diabetes is changing, with more and more people being diagnosed with type 1 diabetes in adulthood, as well as children as young as 8 years old developing type 2 diabetes due to sedentary lifestyles and escalating levels of obesity. As a result, the treatment of diabetes has had to be reconsidered and modified to take into account individual reactions to diabetes and the need to maintain blood glucose levels between 4 and 7 mmol/l at all times, in order to reduce the risk of diabetes-related complications. More recently, in reviewing the link between the incidence of diabetes-related complications and blood glucose control, NICE (2008) has developed guidelines for healthcare practitioners. These suggest setting ideally a target haemoglobin A1c (HbA1c) of no greater than 6.5%, but this needs to be discussed and agreed with the patient. Following on from the discussions with the patient, a higher HbA1c target level may be set if this is what the person wants and is confident that it can be achieved; however achieving and pursuing highly intensive management to achieve HbA1c levels of less than 6.5% should be avoided.

It is no longer possible to predict with accuracy the course of treatment a person will require in order to control their blood glucose levels. While it is accepted that, due to the acute autoimmune response causing type 1 diabetes, the person will require insulin from diagnosis, it also needs to be recognized that this same person may concurrently also require oral antidiabetes medication. Similarly, it is now widely recognized that it is quite probable that a person with type 2 diabetes may require insulin therapy at some stage during the disease process, resulting in an overlap of treatments.

For these reasons, this chapter has been designed to consider the different antidiabetes therapies available, giving suggestions for practice, rather than looking at the possible treatment modalities of type 1 and type 2 diabetes.

Insulin therapy

> The problem of managing diabetes is not the insulin deficiency, but the insulin therapy. (Anon)

A huge array of different forms of insulin, including bovine, porcine and analogue insulin, is currently on the market today. Within each form, manufacturers have created a number of different types, each offering various 'duration of action' times. Deciding on the most appropriate insulin regimen for a person with diabetes can therefore be difficult.

Indications for insulin therapy

The first step in safely navigating this minefield is to determine whether insulin therapy would be an appropriate treatment to be administered on a permanent basis or whether it would be better to be introduced only during acute episodes in a person's life.

The consequences of initiating insulin therapy must be fully understood by healthcare practitioners, as for some people with diabetes it can mean a loss of livelihood. While discrimination against people using insulin is decreasing with the introduction of the Disability Discrimination Act (1995), there are some workplaces where discrimination still exists, e.g. the armed forces are currently exempt from the Disability Discrimination Act and a person with diabetes commencing insulin would be required to leave on medical grounds. Additionally, in the UK people who have larger goods vehicles (LGV) and passenger-carrying vehicle (PCV) driving licenses also have to relinquish their license to the Driver Vehicle Licensing Agency (DVLA) if they commence insulin therapy, which would result in a lorry driver losing his job with potentially serious financial and social consequences.

However, there are times when insulin therapy cannot be avoided, despite the cost to the person's life, and these are listed below.

1. Type 1 diabetes

Type 1 diabetes is associated with autoimmunity, which causes a destruction of beta cells. Approximately 90% of a person's beta cells will have been destroyed before they begin to experience the classic signs and symptoms of diabetes. As mentioned in Chapter 1, this can take a varying length of time depending on the individual, but once a diagnosis of type 1 diabetes has been made it is essential that the person commences on insulin therapy immediately to avoid any serious, life-threatening illness. These people will then require insulin therapy for the rest of their lives.

2. Ketoacidosis

Any person, regardless of their age and type of diabetes, will require insulin therapy to correct an episode of ketoacidosis. Ketoacidosis can rapidly lead to death and therefore needs to be treated promptly and effectively. In the first instance, the insulin therapy will be administered intravenously and generally, although not always, on a 'sliding-scale' regimen. It is given intravenously initially as absorption via this route is much more reliable and consistent than via subcutaneous injections. Once the level of ketoacidosis is reduced and stabilized, the person will then be transferred on to subcutaneous insulin. The cause of the ketoacidosis will determine whether the person needs to continue insulin therapy for the foreseeable future. Further information on the causes and treatment of ketoacidosis can be found in Chapter 3.

3. Failure of diet and oral therapy in type 2 diabetes

Adhering to a healthy diet and lifestyle regimen can help to control blood glucose levels in the initial period for someone with type 2 diabetes; however, diabetes is an insidious condition which never gets better and only gets worse. Over time, people with type 2 diabetes tend to go through an assortment of different combinations of oral therapies but eventually, despite large doses and a range of different antidiabetes tablets, their blood glucose levels will remain high and this puts them at increased risk of serious diabetes complications. In these cases insulin therapy is the final option. It is estimated that after having had type 2 diabetes for 10 years, the majority of people will then require insulin treatment in some shape or form.

4. Intercurrent illness

Anyone with type 2 diabetes who experiences a significant intercurrent illness and is thus unable to control their blood glucose levels and is at risk of developing ketoacidosis will require insulin therapy, at least for the duration of their illness.

5. Pregnancy

Pregnancy and diabetes can be divided into three different categories:

- women who are pregnant and have pre-existing type 1 diabetes,
- women who are pregnant and have pre-existing type 2 diabetes,
- women who develop gestational diabetes during pregnancy.

In the first category, pregnant women with pre-existing type 1 diabetes will already be self-administering insulin. However, insulin requirements change quite dramatically throughout the stages of pregnancy. The Confidential Enquiry into

Maternal and Child Health (2007) reported that in order to reduce the risk of fetal congenital abnormalities and stillbirth, during pregnancy the mother's blood glucose levels should not be higher than 5.5 mmol/l before meals and no higher than 7.7 mmol/l 2 hours after meals. An HbA1c <7% is also required for all women in the preconceptual stage and during pregnancy. In the light of this report, blood glucose levels will need to be monitored very closely and insulin therapy tailored accordingly. Increasingly, this is being done via continuous sub-cutaneous insulin therapy (or insulin pump therapy as it is also known).

Pre-existing type 2 diabetes is a rather new phenomenon. Traditionally, it was people entering old age who were diagnosed as having the equivalent of type 2 diabetes and as such had left behind their child-bearing years. As many younger people are now developing type 2 diabetes, its management during pregnancy needs to be considered. Women taking oral hypoglycaemic agents will need to be commenced on to insulin therapy, ideally preconceptually if the pregnancy is planned and known about, but certainly once pregnancy is confirmed, as many oral hypoglycaemic agents are contraindicated in pregnancy. Once the baby has been delivered and the blood glucose levels stabilize the woman may then recommence her original oral treatment. If she chooses to breast feed, insulin may need to be continued during this time (Confidential Enquiry into Maternal and Child Health 2007).

Gestational diabetes is defined as 'carbohydrate intolerance resulting in hyperglycaemia of variable severity with onset or first recognition during pregnancy' (WHO 1999). It is caused by the action of the placental hormones, which have the effect of increasing the level of insulin resistance, causing blood glucose levels to rise. 'True' gestational diabetes will resolve with the delivery of the placenta and will be confirmed by a normal oral glucose tolerance test (OGTT) 6 weeks postdelivery. An abnormal OGTT at this time indicates that diabetes may have been present, but undetected, prior to the pregnancy.

Gestational diabetes will be treated initially with diet and lifestyle changes; however, it may become necessary to commence insulin in order to keep blood glucose levels within the required levels. Owing to the potential harmful effects of oral antidiabetes medications to the fetus, these should be avoided.

6. Surgery

All patients with both type 1 and type 2 diabetes will require insulin if undergoing major surgery. This will be expected for people already on insulin, but may be a surprise to those who have type 2 diabetes that can be kept under control with diet and lifestyle changes. The physical stress placed on the body during surgery can be significant and the body will deal with this via an increased output of adrenaline, causing an increase in blood glucose levels. Insulin is prescribed in this scenario as its action is more easily and conveniently controlled than oral antidiabetes agents, especially as the body is under stress due to the surgery and the person may need to refrain from eating due to the surgical procedure. It is imperative that blood glucose levels remain within normal limits before, during and after surgery to ensure timely healing of surgical wounds and the prevention of postoperative complications including wound infections (see Chapter 5 for further details and discussion).

Patients with type 2 diabetes requiring minor operations or day surgery generally do not require insulin if they are not currently prescribed it, but their insulin needs should be assessed on an individual basis.

Aim of insulin treatment

When insulin therapy has been initiated and titrated to the individual's needs it should result in:

- Abolition of symptoms such as polyuria, thirst, tiredness, etc. People commencing insulin after a relatively short time comment how much better they feel and report having much more energy.
- Optimization of blood glucose control. The range of insulin preparations currently available ensures that there is a treatment regimen suitable to meet most peoples' needs. It should therefore be possible to prescribe an insulin regimen which, if taken correctly and appropriately, and in addition to diet and lifestyle measures, will maintain blood glucose levels between 4 and 7 mmol/l. However, it is recognized that this is not always easy and may sometimes require input from a specialist team.
- Reduction and prevention of complications. By maintaining blood glucose levels within normal limits and achieving an HbA1c of ≤7.5% the risk of developing diabetes related complications will be significantly reduced. The progression of complications that are already present will also be slowed when blood glucose levels are kept within the target range.
- Maintenance of ideal body weight. Insulin is a growth hormone and has the propensity for weight gain. This needs to be seriously considered for all people requiring insulin therapy but is of particular importance to those with type 2 diabetes who may already be overweight or obese. The aim would be to carefully titrate the insulin amount so that enough is given to control blood glucose levels; however, advice, education and support on diet and lifestyle issues aimed at avoiding weight gain would also need to be provided.

Sources of insulin

Historically, there have been three sources of insulin available for clinical use:

- Bovine – this is insulin removed from an ox pancreas but is rarely used in clinical practice today.
- Porcine – this comes from pig pancreas. The amino acid sequence of pig insulin differs from that of human insulin by only one amino acid sequence, making it highly compatible for use in humans.
- Human – this does not originate from humans but is genetically modified from the bacteria *Escherichia coli* or from the yeast *Saccharomyces crevisiae* as these organisms multiply readily. The majority of people with diabetes now use this type of insulin.

As the administration of human insulin exactly replicates the type of insulin produced naturally in the body, this results in less antibodies being built up against it compared to porcine and bovine insulin. Consequently, it is thought to have a quicker onset and a shorter duration of action than the traditional equivalent animal insulin. It is therefore advisable when transferring a person from animal to human insulin to reduce the initial dose by 10% and to closely monitor the effects of this.

In transferring to human insulin, some people have reported increased difficulty in being able to control their blood glucose levels and their symptoms of impending hypoglycaemia being less pronounced or disappearing altogether. However, when transferred back on to their regular animal insulin, these problems disappear. Unfortunately, the production of animal insulin is in decline with most of the main insulin manufacturing companies discontinuing production in the majority of countries, including the UK. One company, Wockhardt UK, is currently committed to continuing to provide animal insulin for the foreseeable future; however, this may require people to change supplier.

Analogue insulin

Analogue insulin was introduced into the market in the 1990s and is now in widespread use today. Like human insulin, it is synthetic insulin produced by genetic engineering but, unlike human insulin, it does not exactly replicate the insulin that is produced naturally in the beta cells of the pancreas. It can therefore not be labelled 'human insulin' and its correct term is 'analogue insulin'. There are currently four analogue insulins available and used in practice: lispro (Humalog®), aspart (NovoRapid®) detemir (Levemir®) and glargine (Lantus®).

Manufacturing process and the absorption of insulin

The way in which insulin acts once it has been administered can be altered to enable it to have a range of variable onset and duration of action times. Current insulin preparations include short-acting, intermediate-acting, long-acting and peakless long-acting.

Short-acting insulin, e.g. actrapid, is clear in appearance and can be administered subcutaneously or intravenously. It consists of unmodified insulin in a solution that is pH neutral. Once injected subcutaneously, it begins to act 20–30 minutes after injection and has a peak action time of 1–3 hours.

Key point

Actrapid insulin or premixed insulin containing actrapid should *always* be administered at least 30 minutes *before* a meal to enable it to be broken down and at the same time become active as the blood glucose levels begin to rise with the ingestion of food.

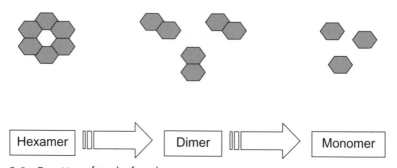

Figure 2.1 Transition of insulin from hexamer to monomer.

Short-acting insulin needs to be given at least 30 minutes before a main meal because the insulin molecules coagulate in the vial to form hexamers (groups of six molecules). These hexamers are too large to be absorbed from the subcutaneous tissues into the circulation and need to be broken down into dimers (groups of two molecules) and ultimately into monomers, which are single insulin molecules (Williams and Pickup 2004) (Figure 2.1). If given 30 minutes before a meal, the peak action time of the short-acting insulin will correspond to the rise in blood glucose levels caused by the food eaten and will prevent hyperglycaemia.

The time of onset of action and duration of action times of insulin can be varied. This is achieved by altering the chemical and pharmacokinetic properties of the insulin by attaching zinc molecules to it. The insulin has to be freed from these attachments at the injection site before absorption into the bloodstream is possible. It is only once the insulin has been absorbed into the bloodstream that it becomes active.

The varying amount of zinc attached to the insulin molecules in the different insulin preparations will determine how long the separation process will take, and therefore how long the duration of action is prolonged. These types of insulin are cloudy in appearance and can only be administered subcutaneously.

Analogue insulin has been modified molecularly so that it works in slightly different ways to the traditional animal or human insulin (Diabetes UK 2006b). Lispro and aspart, which are rapid-acting insulins, have been produced by recombinant technology, whereby two amino acids near to the terminal end of the B chain have been reversed in position. This has resulted in the insulin having a very low tendency to form hexamers, and therefore does not need to be broken down following administration before it becomes active. Reversing the two amino acids does not interfere with the way the insulin is able to bind to the insulin receptor or to its circulating half-life.

The long-acting, peakless analogue insulins, detemir and glargine, have been developed by changing the pH value at which insulin is least soluble and becomes solid. As a result, this type of insulin remains soluble in acidic pH but becomes a solid form when it is injected into the subcutaneous tissues where the pH is near neutral. Thus, the physiological activity of analogue insulin gives a 'flat', 'peak-less' profile (Ahmed 2004).

Main types of insulin

There are six main types of insulin currently available for use in clinical practice:

1. Rapid-acting analogue insulin

As this does not form hexamers and has a peak action at 0–3 hours, it can be injected immediately before, with, or within 20 minutes of eating a meal. This insulin gives the person greater flexibility with their diet and lifestyle. With help and support, the person is able to titrate the number of units of insulin they inject to the amount and type of carbohydrate contained within the meal they are about to eat. Additionally, some people prefer to inject themselves after they have eaten in case they eat less or indeed more than they had originally planned. This method enables them to give the correct amount of insulin accordingly in one injection, and helps to avoid the potential fear of hypoglycaemia as excess insulin for requirements should not, in theory, have been administered.

2. Long-acting analogue

It is advised that this is injected once per day at the same time. This tends to be at the person's bedtime as most people go to bed at the same time each night, thus aiding compliance with the treatment. The time of day in which the injection is given does not generally make any difference, but the important note is that it is given at the same time due to the 24-hour action profile that the insulin has. As it does not have a peak action, it does not need to be given with food.

It is also important to note that traditionally longer-acting human insulin is cloudy in appearance, whereas detemir and glargine are clear. There is, therefore, a risk that the two insulins may be confused. Different insulin pen devices should be given to the patient to help prevent any confusion.

3. Short-acting insulin

This is human insulin that needs to be injected 30 minutes before a meal to ensure that it has broken down from hexamers to monomers in time to cover the rise in blood glucose levels that occur during and after food. It has a peak action of 2–6 hours but can last up to 8 hours, giving rise to the possibility of hypoglycaemia. Once administered, the person needs to ensure that they have adequate diet and nutrition to avoid the occurrence of hypoglycaemia.

4. Medium- and long-acting insulin

These are taken once or twice a day to meet background/basal insulin require-ments. The body requires a small continuous supply of insulin throughout the day and night to provide energy for such things as tissue repair, energy, cellular activity and regeneration. Therefore, if the person is not making any of their own endogenous insulin they will require background insulin for this purpose. These are usually taken in conjunction with a short-acting insulin, which controls the sharp postprandial rise in blood glucose levels.

5. Mixed insulin
This is a factory-produced insulin that combines a medium- and a short-acting insulin together in the same vial.

6. Mixed analogue
This is where a medium-acting insulin has been combined with a rapid-acting analogue insulin.

Common examples of different insulin preparations

Common examples of different insulin preparations are given in Table 2.1.

1. Exubera® – inhaled insulin
Inhaled insulin, Exubera®, was available commercially in the UK until January 2008. Unfortunately, it was then withdrawn due to poor uptake of the drug. It is hoped that, as the technology has now been developed, it may become commercially viable again in the future, giving some people with diabetes a different treatment option.

Inhaled insulin is a rapid-acting human insulin in powder form that has been licensed for use in adults with diabetes. It is inhaled into the lung using a specifically designed handheld inhaler, enabling insulin to be absorbed into the blood

Table 2.1 Examples of different insulin preparations.

	Human	Analogue	Porcine	Bovine
Rapid-acting insulin	–	• NovoRapid® • Humalog® • Apidra®	–	–
Short-acting insulin	• Actrapid® • Humulin® S • Exubera®	–	• Hypurin porcine neutral	• Hypurin bovine neutral
Medium-/ long-acting insulin	• Insulatard® • Humulin® I	–	• Hypurin porcine isophane	• Hypurin bovine isophane
Long-acting insulin	–	• Lantus® • Levemir®	–	–
Mixed insulin	• Mixtard® 30 • Humulin® M3	• NovoMix® 30 • Humalog® Mix 25 • Humalog® Mix 50	• Hypurin porcine 30/70 mix	–

stream via the alveoli. Inhaled insulin is not recommended for the routine treatment of people with type 1 or type 2 diabetes (NICE 2006). However, inhaled insulin may be used as a treatment option for people with type 1 or type 2 diabetes who continue to have poor glycaemic control, despite different therapeutic interventions.

In addition, inhaled insulin can be used when intensive preprandial subcutaneous insulin therapy is not possible, e.g. due to a marked and persistent fear of injections or severe and persistent problems with injection sites (NICE 2006). However, it must be remembered that people with type 1 diabetes cannot have the use of subcutaneous injections totally eradicated by the administration of Exubera®, as the person will still be required to inject an intermediate- or long-acting insulin in combination with the inhaled insulin.

For those patients who meet the NICE (2006) criteria for inhaled insulin, initiation should be carried out within a specialist diabetes centre. Treatment should not be continued beyond 6 months unless there is evidence of a sustained improvement in the person's HbA1c level. In addition, people with diabetes wishing to commence Exubera® must have stopped smoking at least 6 months prior to starting treatment and must not smoke during therapy. Exubera® is contraindicated in people with poorly controlled, unstable or severe asthma, or severe chronic obstructive pulmonary disease and should not be used during pregnancy.

Typical insulin regimens

As people are all individuals with varying eating habits, preferences and lifestyles ranging from being 'sedentary and relaxed' to 'always on the go', it is not possible to adopt a 'one-size fits all' approach to insulin therapy. The range of insulin that is currently available makes it possible and easier to meet individual requirements; however, there are three main insulin regimens that are used typically in practice.

1. Mixed insulin regimen

In this regimen, biphasic or mixed insulin is used. As mentioned previously, this type of insulin contains a mixture of fast-acting insulin, such as actrapid, and intermediate-acting insulin, such as Insulatard®. As this insulin preparation contains actrapid it has to be injected 30 minutes before breakfast and 30 minutes before the evening meal to ensure that it has been broken down and is pharmacologically active as blood glucose levels begin to rise with the ingestion of food. The newer mixed analogue insulin, such as NovoMix® 30 and Humalog® Mix 25, can be given with the first mouthful of food as they do not form hexamers and are broken down immediately.

The number ascribed to the name of the insulin, e.g. Mixtard® 30 and Humalog® Mix 25, refers to the percentage amount of short-acting insulin present in the vial and subsequent dose. Therefore, in Mixtard® 30, 30% of the insulin will be short acting and 70% will be medium acting.

The mechanics of this regimen aim to reduce postprandial blood glucose levels and maintain a small amount of circulating background/basal insulin.

Table 2.2 Action times of Mixtard® 30 insulin and effect on blood glucose levels.

Injection time	Mixtard® 30 – insulin components	Peak onset/ action time	Effect on which blood glucose level
30 min before breakfast	Actrapid®	30 min–3 hours	This works quickly, reducing the rise in blood glucose level following breakfast. Peak action has generally subsided by lunch time.
	Insulatard®	1–12 hours	The peak action of this is increasing throughout the morning and is at a level by mid-day to reduce the lunch-time postprandial rise in blood glucose level. At the same time this insulin provides some basal or background insulin. The main effects become reduced and so do not have a significant effect on the evening meal rise in blood glucose level. A second injection is therefore required.
30 min before evening meal	Actrapid®	30 min–3 hours	As this works quickly is will reduce the postprandial evening meal rise in blood glucose level with the peak action largely subsided by bedtime.
	Insulatard®	1–12 hours	The longer, delayed action of this insulin will provide the person with some insulin for a bedtime snack and with basal insulin throughout the night to provide cellular energy for tissue repair and cell reproduction.

This is achieved by the two different insulin actions complementing each other (Table 2.2).

Difficulties can arise with this regimen as there is an overlap of insulin action times at mid-morning and before bedtime. It is during these times that the person is most at risk of having a hypoglycaemic episode and may require a small mid-morning and bedtime snack to counteract this effect.

2. Basal bolus insulin regimen

This course of treatment is based around two very different insulin preparations – a rapid-acting analogue and a long-acting analogue. The long-acting analogue is a once a day subcutaneous injection, which needs to be given at the same time each day, give or take a maximum of 1 hour. This provides a basal rate of insulin for a 24-hour period. It has a consistent 'flat' profile with no peaks in action, thus making the insulin action reliable and the person less prone to hypoglycaemia. This type of insulin should make up 50% of the person's total daily insulin requirements.

The remaining 50% of the person's total daily insulin will come from a rapid-acting analogue insulin. As this has an almost immediate peak action time and is largely broken down after 2–3 hours, this type of insulin is ideal for reducing postprandial blood glucose levels. It can be given immediately before, during, or within 20 minutes of eating a meal. If the insulin is given prior to eating a meal, the person needs to ensure that they do in fact eat all they planned to and had taken insulin for, in order to avoid hypoglycaemia.

Rapid-acting analogue insulin can also be given as a 'correction dose' between meals if blood glucose levels exceed the normal limits.

Key point

As a rule of thumb, 1 unit of rapid-acting analogue insulin will reduce a person's blood glucose level by 2–3 mmol/l.

---

3. Basal/insulin regimen

This type of regimen involves the use of the long-acting analogue insulin and is used for people who have type 2 diabetes who are having difficulties keeping their baseline blood glucose levels between 4 and 7 mmol/l. The baseline blood glucose levels refer to the amount of glucose in the blood stream first thing in the morning after a natural overnight fast, and from the time 2 hours after they have eaten up to the start of their next main meal.

In general, these people are able to manage the postprandial blood glucose peaks with their own production of insulin, which may be enhanced with different oral therapies. By having one injection per day of the long-acting analogue insulin this can be enough to prevent the overall blood glucose profile from spiralling. This regimen is not suitable for those with type 1 diabetes, as these people require both early (bolus) and late (basal) phase insulin.

Factors to consider when prescribing insulin

When commencing a patient on insulin therapy, or reviewing the treatment of a person who is having difficulty controlling their blood glucose levels, a number of factors need to be considered.

1. How much endogenous insulin is the person producing?

A person who has been diagnosed with type 1 diabetes will be producing very little of their own insulin, and certainly not enough to maintain glucose homeostasis. In these circumstances, this person will need to replace all of their required insulin, which will include their early-phase and late-phase insulin requirements. This person would be best suited to a mixed or basal/bolus insulin regimen.

A person who has type 2 diabetes may be producing some endogenous insulin with the help of oral antidiabetes medication but this is may not be enough to sustain blood glucose levels between 4 and 7 mmol/l. In this scenario, the person may benefit from having some daily, basal insulin being introduced as part of their diabetes treatment therapy. Alternatively, they may be considered for a mixed insulin regimen or even a basal/bolus insulin regimen, depending on their lifestyle and insulin requirements.

2. What sort of lifestyle does the person lead?

Knowing the type of lifestyle a person leads is very important in being able to match the most appropriate insulin regimen to their lifestyle and habits. A person who has quite a lot of 'routine' in their life could be best suited to a mixed insulin regimen. This would mean that they eat similar meals at similar times of the day and their day-to-day level of exercise and activity is relatively constant.

In contrast to this is the person who has a hectic routine, no 2 days are the same in terms of diet and exercise, mealtimes are not regular and at times meals may be delayed or missed. For this person a mixed insulin regimen would not be suitable and would constrict the person too much, therefore a basal-bolus regimen would need to be considered, which will provide added lifestyle flexibility.

3. At what times of the day are the person's blood glucose level well controlled and poorly controlled?

Through the use of regular blood glucose monitoring, it will be possible for the person and healthcare professional to identify patterns and trends in blood glucose control. Different circumstances would dictate which insulin regimen would be the most appropriate. For example, a person with type 2 diabetes experiencing high blood glucose levels first thing in the morning, and although remaining high throughout the day, the levels did rise and fall between meals, may be considered for a basal insulin regimen if maximum oral therapy was not sufficient. As mentioned previously, this would require the person to inject a long-acting analogue insulin such as glargine or detemir once each day, which may be enough to reduce the baseline blood glucose levels and ultimately stabilize them.

Being able to respond appropriately to the above question requires a careful assessment of the individual with diabetes, and for the healthcare professional to have a thorough understanding of the different actions of insulin so that insulin action can be correlated to the person's high and low blood glucose readings.

Case study: Charlotte

Charlotte is a 27-year-old sales representative who was diagnosed with type 1 diabetes at the age of 15 years. Over the years she has managed to gain reasonably good control of her diabetes by giving herself two injections per day of Mixtard® 30 insulin.

Prior to her appointment as a sales representative 6 months ago, she worked as a secretary in a large private business. With her new appointment, her life has become very busy and much less predictable. She is travelling a great deal and is no longer able to have standard meals at regular times of the day; consequently, she is finding it increasingly difficult to control her blood glucose levels and is becoming quite concerned and frustrated.

Discussion of Charlotte's case

At the time when Charlotte was diagnosed with diabetes, mixed insulin regimens were very much common place as basal-bolus insulin regimens were only in the early stages of discovery. She was therefore commenced on the twice daily injections of Mixtard® 30 insulin, which she found to be satisfactory while she was able to control and amend her lifestyle to accommodate the two different insulin actions. Charlotte's lifestyle is now much more hectic and unpredictable; she is not able to eat at the same time each day nor eat a set amount of food, which is required with a mixed insulin regimen. The effects of this, which Charlotte is experiencing, is poor glycaemic control and an increased risk of hypoglycaemia, which is potentially very serious, particularly as she is spending a large proportion of her time driving and therefore needs to avoid hypoglycaemia at all costs.

Charlotte needs to be transferred on to a basal bolus insulin regimen where she will inject her long-acting analogue insulin at night-time, as despite a hectic lifestyle, a person's bedtime tends to remain reasonably static. She will then inject a rapid-acting insulin analogue just before, during, or just after she has eaten, regardless of the time of day. Additionally, if she misses a meal, then she simply does not inject that dose of insulin. This will enable the insulin to be fitted in around her work schedule, rather than the other way round, and she should begin to regain her glycaemic control.

Diet and exercise therapy

1. Diet

Adopting a healthy diet and exercise regimen is crucial for anyone, regardless of whether they have diabetes or not, but for the person with type 2 diabetes, diet and exercise are an essential treatment modality. The aim is for the person to achieve and maintain a healthy body weight, i.e. body mass index (BMI) 18–24 kg/m^2 (Table 2.3). Much research has shown that if a person is able to lose just 10% of their excess body weight this will correspond to a reduction in HbA1c, a lowering of cholesterol levels and a fall in systolic blood pressure (Norris et al. 2004). In addition, any deviation from the recommended 'healthy diet' impacts immediately on raising the person's blood glucose level significantly and thus ultimately impacts on their propensity to develop diabetes-related complications.

Table 2.3 Body mass index (BMI) scale (Chan 2003).

BMI	Classification
<18.5	Underweight/malnutrition
18.5–24.9	Healthy weight
25.0–29.9	Overweight
30.0–39.9	Obese
>40	Morbidly obese

Table 2.4 Glycaemic index (GI) foods (Gallop and Renton 2005).

Glycaemic index rating	Types of food
Low	
Vegetables	Broccoli, cabbage, carrots, cauliflower
Fruit	Apples, pears, oranges, grapefruit, grapes, strawberries
Pasta/bread	Pasta, noodles, wholemeal bread, brown rice
Beans	Baked beans, butter beans, chick peas, red kidney beans
Cereals	Branflakes, porridge oats, muesli
Dairy	Semi-skimmed milk, soya milk cottage cheese, rapeseed oil
Medium	
Vegetables	Yams
Fruit	Apricots, bananas, kiwi, mango, pineapple, sultanas, prunes
Pasta/bread	Potatoes, Indian basmati rice, wholegrain bread, couscous
Beans	—
Cereals/biscuits	Fruit muesli, Fruit and Fibre, digestive biscuits
Dairy	Yoghurt, chocolate, cheese, ice-cream, crème fraiche
High	
Vegetables	Broad beans
Fruit	Melon, raisins, dried fruit, jam, apple puree
Pasta/bread	Tinned pasta and noodles, gnocchi, bagels, white bread
Beans	Baked beans with pork, broad bean, refried beans
Cereals/biscuits	Cornflakes, Frosted Flakes, Sultana Bran, cream crackers
Dairy	Cream cheese, sour milk, cottage cheese, rice milk

The glycaemic index (GI) diet was originally developed as an eating strategy to help a person with diabetes keep their blood glucose levels within normal limits and avoid dramatic blood glucose swings. However, the healthy-eating principles that the diet advocates have also been found to help with weight loss in people who are overweight or obese. The adoption of a low GI diet is recommended and supported by a number of national diabetes associations, who include it within their current dietary guidelines for people with diabetes (Nutrition Subcommittee of the Diabetes Care Advisory Committee of Diabetes UK 2003).

The main principles of this diet are for the person to eat carbohydrates that have been classified as being 'low-GI' (Table 2.4). As absorption of this type of

Table 2.5 Different types of fats (Foster 2004).

Classification of fat	Examples
Saturated	Butter, dripping, meat, full-fat dairy products
Polyunsaturated	Trout, salmon, mackerel, herring
Monounsaturated	Olives, nuts, seeds, avocados, oils from these
Trans fats	Hard margarines, cakes, biscuits

carbohydrate is slower than other carbohydrates, this creates a less spectacular rise in blood glucose level, making diabetes control easier. A feeling a satiety is also generated for a longer period and the person is less inclined to eat frequently or snack, thus ultimately reducing total daily calorie intake. It is important to emphasize that the glycaemic value of carbohydrates needs to be considered alongside sensible portion control. The person is still not free to eat unlimited amounts of low GI carbohydrate foods.

Although the GI diet is principally concerned with carbohydrate intake it is also recommended that fats in the diet (Table 2.5) should be confined to the use of monounsaturated fats, which are produced from nuts, seeds and olives. Lovejoy (2002, cited in Colombani 2004) reported that a diet high in saturated fatty acids, which are generally solid at room temperature and tend to be derived from animal sources, e.g. butter, can have an adverse effect on insulin sensitivity. He concluded that a low-GI diet that was high in monounsaturated fatty acids may actually help to protect against insulin resistance, resulting in improved glycaemic control for the person with diabetes.

2. Exercise

As well as dietary modification, the inclusion of planned, regular exercise into a person's daily routine is required for effective, long-term weight loss and maintenance of blood glucose levels. Walking is an excellent exercise of moderate intensity for people with diabetes and, over time, it will contribute to weigh loss and weight control. It has been found to reduce body fat, decrease insulin resistance and can also improve blood glucose and blood lipid control (Foreyt and Poston 1999).

Regular walking can be incorporated into a person's daily routine relatively simply, but for the person with diabetes specific medical issues and precautions need to be considered. The presence of painful peripheral neuropathy associated with diabetes may make walking more difficult (Albarran *et al.* 2006) and the condition will need to be adequately treated or stabilized before the person can begin exercising regularly. The need for well-fitting shoes should be emphasized to prevent rubbing and the formation of a foot ulcer, as any foot injury in a person with diabetes can have very serious consequences and, if coupled with diabetic neuropathy, may lead to limb amputation.

Table 2.6   Energy expenditure from exercise (Humphries 2002).

Type of exercise	Expenditure/30 min (kcal)
Walking relaxed speed	120
Walking briskly	180
Swimming relaxed speed	255
Cycling leisurely speed	120
Golf	195
House work	120
Gardening, digging	240

For those who are unable to walk at a therapeutic level, any exercise that causes a 40–60% rise in resting heart rate is suitable to enhance weight loss. This may include swimming, cycling, or arm exercises for the person with limited mobility. Table 2.6 gives an estimation of the calories burnt for different types of exercise over a 30-minute period.

In advocating regular exercise, attention needs to be given to the increased risk of experiencing a hypoglycaemic episode during, or up to 15 hours after, exercise. Particularly, patients who are taking a sulphonylurea and/or insulin therapy will need to be educated on the effect their medication and exercise will exert on blood glucose levels if hypoglycaemia is to be avoided.

Tablet therapy

Key point

Tablet therapy *should not* be used as a replacement for diet and exercise therapy – it should be used in combination with both of these.

Tablet therapy should be considered when a person with type 2 diabetes has been unable to obtain adequate glycaemic control at the end of a 3-month trial of intensive diet and exercise modification. However, this may be sooner if the person is becoming unwell due to rising blood glucose levels.

There are a variety of different oral antidiabetes medications available, each working in slightly different ways and exerting different pharmacological effects. Tablet therapy is mainly used for people with type 2 diabetes, but there are occasions when people with type 1 diabetes who are overweight may require tablet therapy as an adjunct to insulin therapy. Equally, it is not unusual for people with type 2 diabetes to be prescribed a cocktail of oral antidiabetes medications, with or without the inclusion of subcutaneous insulin.

> **Key point**
>
> Oral hypoglycaemic agents is a common term used in practice to describe the collection of oral medications used to control blood glucose levels. This is no longer a correct use of terminology, as will be seen, as a number of tablet preparations for diabetes do not cause hypoglycaemia and this is not their intended mode of action.

The decision on which drug(s) to prescribe depends partly on the severity of the symptoms of diabetes the person is experiencing and partly on the person's BMI. Oral antidiabetes medications are divided into different categories:

- sulphonylureas,
- biguanides,
- thiazolidinediones,
- incretin mimetics and incretin enhancers,
- alpha glucosidase inhibitors,
- prandial glucose regulators.

General discussion of each of these classification of drugs and experiences of their use in practice is given in this chapter. Specific doses, indications and contraindications to each of these drugs can be found in the *British National Formulary*, which is regularly updated.

1. Sulphonylureas
Examples

- Chlorpropamide (Diabinese®) – not used very much nowadays as it has a long action time, which increases the risk of hypoglycaemia, especially in the elderly.
- Glibenclamide (Daonil®) – as for chlorpropamide, but the action time is slightly less.
- Gliclazide (Diamicron®) – used widely in current practice.
- Glipizide (Glibenese®, Minodiab®) – used widely in current practice.
- Tolbutamide (Rastinon®) – most suitable for those with renal impairment.
- Glimepiride (Amaryl®) – as for glibenclamide.

This category of drugs was originally developed from sulphonamide antibiotics, which were used in the treatment of typhoid. They were first introduced as a way of treating diabetes in the 1950s, when it was discovered that during the treatment of typhoid these drugs also caused a fall in blood glucose levels.

Action
Sulphonylureas act on the pancreatic beta cells to stimulate insulin secretion, but this will only be effective if there is still sufficient beta-cell function remaining. One argument against the use of sulphonylureas is that there is a requirement to

try and preserve beta-cell function in people with diabetes. In taking this class of drug, the beta cells are required to work much harder, leading to potential exhaustion and ultimate premature death of the cells. Furthermore, in patients who are insulin resistant and already producing copious amounts of insulin naturally, they do not actually need higher levels of insulin to be secreted – this has been shown to exacerbate the insulin resistance. As a result, the use of sulphonylureas in the insulin-resistant people may be more harmful than beneficial.

Indications
Sulphonylureas may also cause weight gain as they lower blood glucose levels, causing the person to feel hungry and therefore to snack more frequently. For this reason they are generally used in non-obese/overweight people, but weight management should still be considered regardless.

Persistent or worsening hyperglycaemia despite sulphonylurea therapy may be an indication of beta-cell failure. In this instance, insulin therapy should be instituted (Bailey and Feher 2004).

Contraindications
Once the tablets have been ingested they will increase insulin production, regardless of whether the patient has eaten or not. Therefore, there is an increased risk of hypoglycaemia, particularly when meals are delayed, missed, smaller than usual, and/or the person is more active than usual.

2. Biguianides
Examples
Metformin is the only biguanide drug currently available on prescription. It was introduced as a treatment for diabetes in the 1960s, along with phenformin and buformin. However, phenformin and buformin were withdrawn from most countries in the 1970s as there was a high incidence of lactic acidosis when these drugs were used (Bailey and Feher 2004).

Action
Rather than lowering blood glucose levels, like the sulphonylureas, metformin acts to prevent a rise in hyperglycaemia and consequently does not lower plasma glucose concentrations. It is also not dependent on the presence of functioning pancreatic beta cells, as are the sulphonylureas (Katzung 1998). The main way in which it controls blood glucose levels is by reducing the amount of glucose the liver produces and reducing the amount of glycogen the liver breaks down and releases into the circulatory system. It is also thought that metformin slows down the absorption of glucose from the gastrointestinal tract, thus delaying and reducing the peak in blood glucose levels postprandially (Katzung 1998).

Metformin also acts by promoting the recycling of insulin receptors on to the surface of target cells, which in turn increases the amount of glucose that is able to enter the cells from the blood stream (Galbraith *et al.* 1999). This is an enormous pharmacological help in those people who have type 2 diabetes and are insulin resistant and as a consequence have a reduced number of insulin receptors.

> **Key point**
>
> When taken on its own, metformin *does not* cause hypoglycaemia or weight gain.

Indications
Metformin is the drug of choice in people who have type 2 diabetes and are overweight or obese and therefore have a degree of insulin resistance. In prescribing metformin, the main aim is to enhance the action of the insulin a person is producing naturally or is injecting subcutaneously, thereby resulting in the need for less insulin to maintain normoglycaemia.

It can be used in combination with insulin and other antidiabetes medications such as sulphonylureas and thiazolidinediones and is being used more frequently in people who have type 1 diabetes and are insulin resistant.

The Diabetes Prevention Programme (DPP) (Knowler *et al*. 2002) found that when metformin was prescribed in people who were classified obese and at high risk of developing diabetes, the onset of diabetes could be delayed or even prevented in 31% of the sample, compared to those taking a placebo (Knowler *et al*. 2002). However, the DPP also found that by complying with a healthy lifestyle intervention without the use of metformin, the incidence of diabetes could be delayed or prevented in 58% of the sample population.

Contraindications
Metformin is contraindicated in people with renal disease, alcoholism and hepatic disease, as there is an increased risk of lactic acidosis developing when used in the presence of these diseases.

The gastrointestinal side-effects of metformin are common, occurring in up to 20% of people prescribed the drug. They include anorexia, nausea, vomiting, abdominal discomfort and diarrhoea. The incidence of side-effects tends to be dose related, therefore when commencing metformin it is advised to start with a low dose of 500 mg/day and, if tolerated, very gradually increase the dose to a maximum of 3000 mg/day, or until normoglycaemia is achieved. Alternatively, slow-release metformin can be prescribed which may help to alleviate the unpleasant side-effects.

3. Thiazolidinediones
Examples
Also known as 'glitazones', rosiglitazone and pioglitazone are the two drugs currently available in this category. Since 2000, they have been widely available for the treatment of people with type 2 diabetes as either a first-line monotherapy or as a second-line dual therapy.

Action
These drugs target insulin resistance by increasing the action of the circulating insulin, which in turn increases glucose uptake by the target cells. Glucose oxidation in both muscle and adipose tissue is also increased and hepatic glucose output is decreased. In addition, thiazolidinediones increase lipogenesis and decrease the amount of fatty acids that are released into the circulation (Bailey and Feher 2004), all of which help to reduce plasma glucose levels.

Indications
These drugs are an ideal choice for people who are overweight or obese and have type 2 diabetes, as their main action is to increase insulin sensitivity resulting in less insulin production being required to generate normal blood glucose levels. They are particularly useful for people who are unable to tolerate metformin and as their actions are similar to, but not the same as, metformin they can be used in combination with other antidiabetes agents, including insulin. Indeed, rosiglitazone is now produced in two fixed-dose combinations with either metformin, known as Avandamet®, or with glimepiride, known as Avandaryl®.

Contraindications
Original licensing approval of rosiglitazone was given based on the drug's ability to reduce blood glucose levels and HbA1c levels. However, initial studies were not specifically designed and undertaken to determine the effects of this agent on microvascular and macrovascular complications of diabetes, including cardiovascular morbidity and mortality (Centre for Drug Evaluation and Research 1999). In an extensive literature search that included the website of the Food and Drug Administration and a clinical trials registry maintained by the drug manufacturer GlaxoSmith, Nissen and Wolski (2007) concluded that rosiglitazone was associated with a significant increase in the risk of myocardial infarction and with an increase in the risk of death from cardiovascular causes that had borderline significance. As a result, patients and healthcare professionals should consider the potential for serious adverse cardiovascular effects of treatment with rosiglitazone for type 2 diabetes and patients be given the option of changing treatment to pioglitazone.

Regardless of the research findings of Nissen and Wolski (2007), patients with hepatic impairment, hepatic disease or have a history of congestive cardiac failure should not be prescribed these drugs.

Side-effects of these drugs include significant weight gain, fluid retention and anaemia. Therefore, the patient needs to be monitored closely for the presence of these unwanted side-effects and should be supported in efforts to maintain their current weight or indeed achieve some weight loss if required.

4. Incretin mimetics and incretin enhancer
Examples

- Incretin mimetics – exenatide (Byetta®).
- Incretin enhancer – sitagliptin (Januvia®).

These two types of drugs offer a very new and different approach to the treatment of type 2 diabetes. Their pharmacological activity targets the gastrointestinal tract, rather than the pancreas and insulin secretion directly.

Exenatide was first discovered during a search for biologically active peptides in lizard venom and, after extensive research trialling, its effect on lowering blood glucose levels was approved in April 2005 by the US Food and Drug Administration for the treatment of type 2 diabetes. Subsequently, it has been approved for use in Europe and is being prescribed to patients whose type 2 diabetes is not well controlled on oral agents.

Sitagliptin was first launched on to the pharmaceutical market in July 2006 and the UK became the first European country to access and prescribe this new class of agent in April 2007.

Action
In all people, the simple ingestion of food triggers a complex secretory effect in which multiple gastrointestinal incretin hormones are released. These hormones aid the regulation of gut motility, secretion of gastric acid and pancreatic enzymes, as well as controlling gall bladder contractions and the absorption of nutrients. Incretin hormones also stimulate the secretion of insulin from the beta cells of the pancreas (Drucker and Nauck 2006).

Incretin hormones are defined as hypoglycaemic-inducing hormones and, while there are a number of gastrointestinal hormones that exert different levels of incretin activity, the principle incretin hormones linked to blood glucose regulation are glucose-dependent insulinotropic polypeptide (GIP) and glucagon-like peptide-1 (GLP-1). GIP hormones are secreted from K cells in the duodenum and upper jejunum, whereas GLP-1 is secreted from the L cells in the distal ileum (Campbell and Day 2007).

These two hormones have been found to have a substantial role in reducing blood glucose levels. GLP-1, in particular, does this by reducing glucagon secretion, increasing the feeling of satiety and slowing gastric emptying. In addition, it has been found to improve myocardial function and increase cardiac output (Drucker 2007).

In people with type 2 diabetes, the activity of GIP appears to be reduced and while the incretin activity of GLP-1 is generally retained, the levels of GLP-1 are reduced (Campbell and Day 2007). Additionally, GLP-1 is rapidly degraded by the enzyme dipeptidyl peptidase-4 inhibitor (DPP-4) within 2 minutes of being secreted, leading to a decreased hypoglycaemic effect on blood glucose levels.

In efforts to counteract these negative aspects of blood glucose control, pharmaceutical companies have developed incretin mimetics and incretin enhancers. Exenatide is given by injection and mimics many of the actions of GLP-1, allowing the body to respond to blood glucose changes as they occur. Sitagliptin is taken orally and aims to inhibit the action of DPP-4, thus increasing the circulating levels of GLP-1. Both of these drugs endeavour to decrease blood glucose levels without causing hypoglycaemia.

Indications
Both incretin mimetics and incretin enhancers have been developed for use in people with type 2 diabetes. They have been shown to improve postprandial blood glucose readings and lower HbA1c levels (Aschner *et al.* 2006). As they do not increase insulin secretion *per se*, there is no risk of the person becoming hypoglycaemic when they are taken as a monotherapy or with metformin, rosiglitazone or pioglitazone.

Exenatide and sitagliptin are also indicated as adjunct therapy to improve glycaemic control in those with type 2 diabetes who are already taking metformin, a sulphonylurea, a thiazolidinedione, or a combination of the above, but have not been able to achieve adequate glycaemic control.

Exenatide has also been associated with weight loss (DeFronzo *et al.* 2005), which is an added pharmacological benefit of the drug for many people with type 2 diabetes. This advantage over sitagliptin, which is weight neutral, may help to lessen the disadvantage of having to inject exenatide each day.

Nathan *et al.* (2006) recommend the commencement of metformin at the time of diagnosis for people with type 2 diabetes, with treatment being rapidly intensified until an HbA1c ≤7% is achieved. Sitagliptin offers another alternative as the initial add-on agent and offers greater benefit to blood glucose control when used early in the disease process.

Contraindications
Exenatide is not recommended for use in type 1 diabetes or in patients with type 2 diabetes who have severe renal impairment or end-stage renal disease. As it causes delayed gastric emptying, it should be avoided in people with severe gastrointestinal disease and it may delay the rate of absorption of other drugs being taken. Medications that are dependent on threshold concentrations for efficacy, such as oral contraceptives and antibiotics, should be taken at least 1 hour before the exenatide injection.

Approximately 79% of sitagliptin is excreted unchanged in the urine at a rate of ~350 ml/min therefore it should not be used in patients with moderate or severe renal insufficiency, classified as a creatinine clearance <50 ml/min (Campbell and Day 2007). As there is currently a lack of research into the efficacy of sitagliptin in other categories, it should not be used in children under the age of 18 years and only used with caution in those aged over 75 years. Sitagliptin has been detected in clinically relevant amounts in the milk of lactating animals and for this reason should not be used during pregnancy or breast feeding.

Both drugs are generally tolerated well, but some patients complain of nausea, abdominal pain and diarrhoea. These undesirable effects tend to lessen and disappear over time and generally have not been found significant enough to force discontinuation of treatment.

5. Alpha glucosidase inhibitors
Examples
The only member of this class of drug used in the UK is acarbose, which was introduced into clinical practice in 1991. However, the limited efficacy, cost and

gastrointestinal side-effects associated with this drug have restricted its use in the UK.

Action

The aim of acarbose is to lower postprandial hyperglycaemia by slowing down the rate at which carbohydrates are digested in the gastrointestinal tract. By doing this, the body is not subjected to a sudden sharp rise in postprandial blood glucose levels and therefore does not require a substantial amount of insulin to be released in order to return the rising blood glucose levels back to within normal limits. By reducing the amount of insulin that is required, it is hoped that a person with type 2 diabetes will be able to produce enough of their own endogenous insulin to cope with the delayed and less-dramatic rise in blood glucose levels.

The effectiveness of acarbose is dependent on it being taken together with a meal that is rich in complex carbohydrates, such as that advocated in the GI diet. Patient education in choosing the correct foods and compliance with a healthy diet are therefore essential when acarbose is prescribed.

Indications

This drug is used to control postprandial glycaemic peaks in people with type 2 diabetes who may, or may not be, overweight or obese. It does not have a thera-peutically significant effect on a person's basal blood glucose level. However, as mentioned previously, the effects of this drug are generally modest to poor and therefore acarbose is not commonly prescribed in clinical practice.

Contraindications

Acarbose should not be prescribed in people who have severe renal or liver disease or have a history of chronic intestinal disorders. As long as these contraindications are respected then acarbose has a satisfactory safety record and, significantly, does not cause hypoglycaemia (Bailey and Feher 2004).

6. Meglitinides

Examples

These are also known as prandial glucose regulators. Repaglinide, introduced in 1998, and nateglinide, available for use since 2001, are the two drugs within this category currently available in the UK. Both are rapid-acting and short-acting insulin releasers.

Action

These drugs work in a similar way to sulphonylureas in that they require adequate beta-cell function to enable increased amounts of insulin to be secreted. The difference with these drugs, compared to sulphonylureas, is that they have a faster onset of action and are very short acting, thus reducing the incidence of hypoglycaemia.

The aim of these drugs is to cause a rapid stimulation of insulin secretion at the beginning of meal digestion, which mimics the acute 'early' phase of insulin secretion that occurs naturally in people who do not have diabetes. The effect of the surge of insulin to the liver also helps to suppress hepatic glucose production. This results in reduced postprandial rises in blood glucose levels.

Indications

Meglitinides can be used as a first-line monotherapy in the treatment of non-obese and obese people with type 2 diabetes, in particular those people who are susceptible to postprandial blood glucose peaks. They can also be taken in combination with metformin, acarbose, insulin and thiazolidinediones; however, these drugs tend to be more expensive than conventional sulphonylurea therapy and experience in practice has shown limited effects on reducing blood glucose levels.

As meglitinides are rapidly absorbed, reaching a maximum plasma concentration within 1 hour, the risk of hypoglycaemia is reduced; however, they need to be taken with food. If the patient does not eat, they do not take the drug. To ascertain the efficiency of the drug and the appropriate dose, blood glucose levels should be recorded 2 hours after each meal, by which time it is expected that they should have returned to within normal limits.

Contraindications

These drugs are contraindicated in the treatment of type 1 diabetes as they rely on a degree of functioning beta cells that is absent in type 1 diabetes. They should be avoided in people with severe hepatic impairment or those who have a hypersensitivity to any of the drug components. They are also not recommended in pregnancy, during breast feeding or in children, as clinical trials have not been conducted to establish the safety of these drugs in these groups (Bailey and Feher 2004).

Case study: David

David is a 52-year-old man working full time as a long-distance lorry driver. He was diagnosed with type 2 diabetes 4 months ago. Since the diagnosis was made, he has seen a dietitian to discuss his diet and lifestyle and a healthy eating plan was devised, which he was asked to follow for a period of 3 months. No oral medication was prescribed at this time.

David has a very irregular pattern to his working day and eats at very different times of the day and night, often snacking on chocolate, cakes, crisps and biscuits. As a result he is overweight with a BMI of 32 kg/m^2 and a waist circumference of 102 cm. Owing to his variable working pattern, which includes days and nights away from home, he finds fitting in planned exercise very difficult.

Following a 3-month trial of diet and lifestyle changes, David returns to see his general practitioner (GP), who repeats the HbA1c blood test. The results show an HbA1c of 8.9% indicating that David's blood glucose control needs to be improved significantly if he is to limit his risk of developing diabetes-related complications.

Discussion of David's case

Given the issues relating to David's lifestyle and the fact that his BMI is within the obese category, it is highly likely that a large proportion of David's diabetes is due to insulin resistance. As diet, exercise and lifestyle changes have not improved his blood glucose levels significantly, the GP needs to consider introducing some oral medication.

The drug of choice in this situation would be metformin, with or without a thiazolidinedione such as pioglitazone. This will help reduce the insulin resistance and therefore enable the currently circulating insulin to exert an increased effect on blood glucose levels. As metformin is not always well tolerated, a low dose of 500 mg per day would be commenced, gradually increasing it if tolerated gastrointestinally.

As David's lifestyle is far from conventional and his eating patterns are erratic, sulphonylureas should be avoided, as they require the person to eat at similar times of each day and to have similar-sized meals of similar composition to avoid the incidence of hypoglycaemia. Additionally, as David drives for a living, hypoglycaemia should be avoided at all costs and he will need to inform the DVLA that he has diabetes, which is being treated with tablets. Should he require insulin at a later date, he will need to inform the DVLA of the change in treatment and this may mean that his driving licence is withdrawn.

As this treatment is being considered early in the disease process, it would also be appropriate to prescribe David an incretin mimetic or an incretin enhancer. It is expected that upon explanation to David, sitagliptin would be preferred instead of exenatide, as it can be taken orally. These would aid in the secretion of insulin postprandially without causing hypoglycaemia.

This treatment regimen should be followed for a period of 6 months, at the end of which a repeat HbA1c would be performed. The doses of oral medication can then be reviewed and doses titrated until satisfactory blood glucose control is achieved.

As diabetes is an insidious, progressive disease, long-term blood glucose control needs to be monitored on a 6–12-month basis with metformin doses and other oral antidiabetes medications being tried. However, if after a period of time satisfactory blood glucose control cannot be achieved, evidenced by HbA1c levels >7.5%, then insulin therapy may need to be introduced, either as a monotherapy or in conjunction with metformin and/or a thiazolidinedione.

Conclusion

This chapter has considered the different treatment options available to people with diabetes when trying to create a state of normoglycaemia. Different types of insulin and insulin regimens have been discussed, as well as the range of oral antidiabetes agents and their use in different clinical situations. However, the importance of a healthy diet and planned and regular exercise cannot be underestimated as an effective treatment for diabetes.

Treating diabetes effectively is largely about 'educated trial and error'. What may be very effective in one person may not exhort the desired effect in another. It is therefore vitally important that the healthcare team providing care for people with diabetes fully understand the actions and mechanics of the different antidiabetes medications and are able to match these as close as possible to the person's dietary and lifestyle habits.

Throughout this book, the treatment of diabetes and a range of different problems encountered by people trying to control their diabetes will be explored in the case studies which are presented in each chapter.

Further information

Further information on the different insulin preparations currently available commercially can be found on the following websites:

Lilly	http://www.lilly.co.uk
Novo Nordisk	http://www.novonordisk.co.uk
Pfizer	http://www.pfizer.co.uk
Sanofi-Aventis	http://www.sanofi-aventis.co.uk
Wockhardt UK	http://www.wockhardt.co.uk

Additional information on commercially available insulin can also be found at http://www.diabetes.org.uk/Documents/Magazines/Insulinwallchart.pdf.

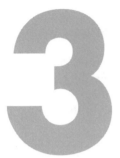

Management and treatment of acute diabetes complications in Accident and Emergency

Aims of the chapter

This chapter will:

1. Identify and discuss the pathophysiological changes that occur in the body as a result of hyperglycaemia and hypoglycaemia.
2. Discuss a range of factors that may cause blood glucose levels to become higher or lower than the accepted normal range of 4–7 mmol/l.
3. Critically consider the immediate and acute management required to return blood glucose levels to within normal limits.

The focus of this chapter is based on two case studies that are used to discuss the treatment, management and care given to two different people attending an Accident and Emergency unit; one person is experiencing hyperglycaemia and diabetic ketoacidosis and the other person has developed hypoglycaemia. However, the management and care described in the chapter can also be applied to any person with diabetes who experiences these complications, regardless of the care setting.

Hyperglycaemia and diabetic ketoacidosis

Definitions

Hyperglycaemia is the term used to describe a blood glucose level >10 mmol/l, regardless of whether the person has any accompanying signs and symptoms. In many cases the symptoms associated with hyperglycaemia do not usually occur until the blood glucose level is persistently >15 mmol/l. The person may then complain of polyuria, polydipsia, weight loss, blurred vision, abdominal pain, weakness and vomiting, which include the signs and symptoms of someone with newly diagnosed diabetes as discussed Chapter 1. These symptoms are a result of the body's compensatory mechanism to reduce the level of acidosis and try to return the blood glucose levels to within normal limits.

Diabetic ketoacidosis (DKA) can result from untreated hyperglycaemia and is a life-threatening complication of diabetes. Significant numbers of people with diabetes are admitted to hospital each year as a consequence of developing DKA. As the number of people developing diabetes rises, an increase in the number of people with diabetes who develop DKA is expected.

DKA is due to a relative or absolute deficiency of insulin. It is the most common hyperglycaemic emergency in patients with diabetes (Umpierrez *et al.* 2004), with the patient often needing management in an intensive care unit due to the level of monitoring required (Savage and Kilvert 2006). In fact, there is evidence to suggest that clinical outcomes are improved when the patient is managed by a diabetes specialist team, rather than by a general physician (Levetan *et al.* 1999) but unfortunately this is not always possible. As a result, many hospitals have developed local guidelines for the treatment of diabetes-related emergencies in an attempt to provide consistent and high-quality care and management. Despite the development of local guidelines and protocols, a 3.4–4.6% mortality rate due to DKA persists (Wallace *et al.* 2001). Mortality is most likely to occur if there is an underlying serious intercurrent illness or if the DKA is misdiagnosed, untreated or undertreated (Ilag *et al.* 2003).

DKA occurs predominantly in people with type 1 diabetes but has also been known to develop in people with type 2 diabetes who have developed a severe infection or are experiencing metabolic stress. Rodacki *et al.* (2007) conducted a study examining the effects of ethnicity and age on the frequency of DKA at the onset of type 1 diabetes. They found that the development of DKA was higher in non-white patients, mainly those from Afro-Caribbean descendants, suggesting that this could indicate a peculiar characteristic of type 1 diabetes in this cohort. They also reported that the development of DKA at onset of diabetes was more prevalent in children up to the age of 10 years, signifying a more aggressive destruction of the beta cells resulting in more sudden and severe clinical presentations in those diagnosed with diabetes at an early age.

Pathophysiology of DKA

DKA mainly arises as a result of a reduction in effective concentrations of circulating insulin and an associated rise in counter-regulatory hormones such as catecholamines, glucagon, growth hormone and cortisol. These hormonal alterations result in the development of three major metabolic events: (1) hyperglycaemia; (2) an increase in the breakdown of protein molecules; and (3) increased lipolysis and ketone production.

1. Hyperglycaemia
The rise in blood glucose level that typifies DKA is due to a decrease in insulin secretion and glucose utilization. As discussed in Chapter 1, the presence of

circulating insulin 'unlocks' target cells and enables glucose to be transported from the blood stream into the liver, muscle cells and adipose tissue, thus reducing the overall blood glucose level. At the same time, insulin also enables the effective utilization of glucose for energy. If there are insufficient amounts of active, circulating insulin, hyperglycaemia will result.

Hyperglycaemia initially causes the movement of water and potassium out of cells, which eventually causes intracellular dehydration and hypokalaemia, expansion of extracellular fluid and a loss of sodium. It also leads to increased diuresis and polyuria, resulting in dehydration and volume depletion causing a diminished urine production and flow and a greater retention of glucose in the plasma. Eventually, metabolic acidosis will occur (Kitabchi and Wall 1999). Glycosuria will also be evident once the blood glucose levels exceed the person's individual renal threshold.

2. Increase in the breakdown of protein molecules

Insulin deficiency and the relative glucagon excess also generate an increase in the breakdown of protein into the constituent amino acids, which are subsequently converted into energy. This is in response to the body not being able to obtain energy supplies from the usual glucose source. This results in amino acidaemia, which causes a detrimental increase in the level of gluconeogenesis with the liver absorbing the amino acids and converting them to glucose, thus worsening the hyperglycaemia and the ensuing diuresis.

3. Increased lipolysis and ketone production

Although there is an abundance of glucose in the blood stream, this is unable to enter the cells due to the absence of insulin. The alpha cells in the Islets of Langerhans of the pancreas are able to detect low intracellular glucose levels and respond to this by secreting glucagon. The alpha cells are not able to identify high blood glucose levels so they respond in the way they do to try to increase the intracellular glucose levels. Unfortunately, the problems of hyperglycaemia are compounded by the action of the alpha cells.

The secretion of glucagon stimulates the liver to release glucose from its reserve supply of glycogen and at the same time adrenaline, cortisol and growth hormones are also released in an attempt to provide the body with energy. The release of these hormones further decreases the effectiveness of any circulating insulin (Gillespie and Campbell 2002). Once the supplies of glycogen have been exhausted the body then begins to break down triglycerides into their constituent fatty acids, which are converted by the liver into the ketones acetoacetate and beta-hydroxybutyrate, for energy. Ketones are excreted via the kidneys and can be detected in urine; however, when production of ketone bodies exceeds excretion this can cause significant, life-threatening acidosis (Kettyle and Arky 1998).

It is worth noting that ketoacidosis tends to be a complication of type 1 diabetes, as people with type 2 diabetes generally have enough active circulating insulin to restrain and prevent ketosis (Kettyle and Arky 1998).

Case study: Pippa

Pippa is a 16-year-old girl who is brought into Accident and Emergency one morning by her mother, who is becoming increasingly worried about her daughter's condition. During the past 2 days she has developed unexplained abdominal pain and leg cramps and has been feeling nauseous and is vomiting 4–5 times per day. Pippa also complains of feeling tired, lethargic and 'washed out' but thinks that this is related to the nausea and vomiting and the fact that she is under increasing amounts of stress at the moment as she is currently sitting her school examinations. She also mentions that she has had blurred vision at times during the past 2 weeks and has been feeling thirsty and needing to pass large amounts of urine more frequently. Her mother has also noticed that Pippa appears to be losing weight, as her clothes are becoming too big for her.

Past medical history

- Appendix removed aged 8 years.

Family history

- Full-time school girl.
- Does not drink alcohol, smoke or take drugs.
- Slim build.
- Member of the school swimming and hockey teams.
- Mother aged 52 years, alive and well, works as a secretary in a local building firm.
- Father aged 54 years, alive and well, works as a postman.
- Pippa has one younger brother aged 13 years, who is fit with no health concerns.
- Both sets of grandparents who are in their 70s are still alive and not suffering from any major illnesses.
- No family history of heart disease, stroke, diabetes, hypertension, thyroid disease or epilepsy.

Medication

- No regular medication.

Allergies

- Penicillin.

Examination

- Semi-conscious.
- Abdomen tender and distended.

- Vomiting bile-stained fluid.
- Not tolerating oral diet or fluids.
- Blood pressure   100/60 mmHg.
- Pulse   136 bpm, regular.
- Temperature   36.1°C.
- Respirations   24/minute.
- Capillary blood glucose level   32.7 mmol/l.
- Venous blood glucose level   38.4 mmol/l.
- Venous bicarbonate   9 mmol/l.
- Potassium   5.0 mmol/l.
- Urinary ketones   ++++.
- HbA1c   7.9%.

Discussion of Pippa's case

In considering the assessment and biochemical information that has been obtained from Pippa and her mother, it becomes apparent that she is experiencing an episode of DKA, potentially relating to a new diagnosis of diabetes. The acute history that she gives of developing symptoms over 2 days provides an indication of type 1 diabetes which classically, but certainly not exclusively, occurs in teenagers and is of sudden onset. She also complains of the typical signs and symptoms of diabetes including tiredness, lethargy, weight loss, thirst and polyuria. Her past medical and family history does not reveal any specific items of note.

As Pippa has not been diagnosed with diabetes previously and there is no history of diabetes in the family, this may account for the reason why she is unable to link the nausea and vomiting to another cause. Vomiting is a common feature of ketoacidosis and is associated with a loss of sodium from the gastrointestinal tract (Hand 2000).

1. Vital signs
Her vital signs are cognisant of DKA, her pulse rate indicates tachycardia resulting from the increased secretion of adrenaline and stress hormones and her temperature is within normal limits, which enables an underlying infection to be ruled out.

She is tachypnoeic and her breath will smell of acetone or pear drops, another common sign of DKA. This occurs as a result of the body's defence mechanism to try and reduce the level of acidosis via respiratory excretion. Finally, her blood pressure is currently within normal parameters but will need to be monitored as increasing dehydration can cause it to drop. Patients with DKA can have on average a deficit of 5–7 litres of fluid.

2. Biochemical markers
The biochemical results further assist in confirming the diagnosis of DKA. As would be expected, Pippa has raised capillary and venous blood glucose levels.

While hand-held blood glucose machines have an excellent accuracy record when the blood glucose levels are within normal limits or thereabouts, the more out of target range a blood glucose is, the less reliable the hand-held glucose meter reading becomes. It is also imperative that venous blood glucose samples, once taken, are sent to the laboratory quickly as blood glucose levels in the sample deteriorate over time, giving unreliable results.

Pippa's venous bicarbonate analysis gives an indication to the level of acidosis. The normal pH of blood is 7.35–7.45, which is predominantly maintained by the bicarbonate buffer system. If acids accumulate in the blood, this causes an increase in hydrogen ion concentration. Bicarbonate is able to neutralize hydrogen ions by incorporating them into water. However, if the hydrogen ion concentration continues to rise, bicarbonate levels are not sufficient to maintain the blood pH. Bicarbonate levels can easily be measured via a heparinized arterial blood sample (Hand 2000).

Pippa has positive levels of ketones in her urine. Different methods have been developed to monitor ketone bodies, including urinary dipsticks, laboratory quantitative readings and hand-held monitors, which use capillary blood to measure levels of 3-beta-hydroxybyturate (3HB). During periods of insulin deprivation and rising blood glucose levels, 3HB is the dominating ketone body produced in the liver. As treatment for DKA is initiated, 3HB is converted to acetoacetate, the substance that is detected when measuring ketones using a urinary dipstick (Henriksen *et al.* 2006). Based on this knowledge, the American Diabetes Association (2005a) have concluded that it is not appropriate to use urine measurements for ketone bodies to diagnose or monitor the course of DKA, as they only provide a retrospective indication of the person's metabolic state. Pippa therefore needs to have her blood ketone levels assessed and monitored and the results recorded.

Although Pippa has a potassium level at the upper end of normal, this does not give an accurate representation of the total body potassium levels which will *always* be markedly depleted, with a deficit ranging between 3 and 12 mmol/kg (Page and Hall 1999). This has the potential of causing fatal cardiac arrhythmias and consequently needs to be corrected immediately and carefully monitored.

Pippa's haemoglobin A1c (HbA1c) is also raised. While this is not, and should not be, used to diagnose DKA, it gives an indication that she has been having high blood glucose readings for a period of time, which helps to make a diagnosis of diabetes more likely. Indeed for many people, ketoacidosis is the main initial presenting event of diabetes mellitus.

Diagnosing DKA

Diagnosing DKA is not difficult, but the combination of high blood glucose levels, acidosis and ketones must be present in order to rule out other conditions causing acidosis, such as salicylate overdose, sepsis or lactic acidosis.

The classical signs and symptoms are those displayed by Pippa in the case study, but if treatment for DKA is delayed then the body eventually decompensates, which causes the person to develop:

- warm dry skin,
- hypothermia,
- hypoxia and a decreased conscious state,
- decreased renal output,
- decreased respirations,
- bradycardia.

Causes of DKA

There are a number of causes that need to be considered in the development of DKA.

1. Lack of insulin

In Pippa's case this is the main cause of her DKA. Owing to autoimmunity, her beta cells have become progressively destroyed, resulting in the levels of circulating insulin becoming diminished. As she has not been diagnosed with diabetes previously, she has not been receiving any treatment for this and as a result her blood glucose levels have begun to rise uncontrollably. She complains of developing symptoms over a 2-week period, indicating quite a quick onset which is typical, although not exclusive, in type 1 diabetes.

People who are known to have diabetes and are being treated with insulin can also develop DKA if: (1) an insulin dose has been forgotten or purposefully omitted; (2) they have given themselves subcutaneous insulin but the number of units is too small to meet their requirements; (3) some of the insulin injected has 'leaked' out of the injection site, resulting in a smaller than planned dose being absorbed, which is difficult to recalculate; and/or (4) they have injected the insulin into a lipohypertrophic lump, which may cause the insulin to be absorbed erratically.

2. Lack of oral hypoglycaemic medication, or failure to respond effectively to it

This can happen if the person with diabetes is prescribed tablets from the sulphonylurea and/or prandial glucose regulator groups of medication, which act by stimulating an increased insulin release. Forgetting to take the prescribed medication at the correct time or if the medication is vomited back or passes through the gastrointestinal tract too quickly can cause insulin deficiency resulting in DKA.

3. Increased amount of food

If the prescribed insulin or oral hypoglycaemic medication is not sufficient to cope with the rising blood glucose levels resulting from food intake, then the person is at an increased risk of developing DKA.

Classically, many people with diabetes will point to birthdays, Christmas, holidays and family celebrations as being the cause of hyperglycaemia, with or without resulting DKA. For most of the time, their daily insulin requirements and blood glucose levels can be adequately controlled but are not augmented to deal with the increased number of calories consumed during these high times and holidays.

4. Reduced amount of exercise

Regular exercise plays an important role in helping to reduce blood glucose levels. The amount and duration of exercise a person with diabetes takes needs to be factored into their decisions regarding the effect it will have on their blood glucose levels and therefore how much insulin they need to inject. Someone who plans to undertake strenuous exercise should reduce their insulin levels accordingly to prevent hypoglycaemia, but in doing this they need to make sure that they do actually undertake the planned amount of exercise. Failure to do so will result in not enough insulin being given, leading to hyperglycaemia and, if left untreated, DKA.

5. Infection and myocardial infarction

Infections, particularly of the gastrointestinal and urinary tracts, and myocardial infarction can stimulate the release of stress-responding hormones such as adrenaline, which antagonize the effects of insulin and result in hyperglycaemia and DKA (Kettyle and Arky 1998). Therefore, a person with type 1 diabetes who is admitted to hospital due to DKA would need to be assessed for the presence of an underlying infection or myocardial infarction. It must be remembered that the presence of diabetic neuropathy, a common complication of diabetes, may mask the symptoms of an acute infection or inflammatory process, making diagnosis much more difficult.

6. Injury

As with infection, any injury or trauma that may lead to the release of stress hormones increases the risk of the person with diabetes developing DKA.

7. Menstruation

Many women with diabetes have commented that they notice an increase in their blood glucose levels a few days before their menstrual period begins (Lunt and Brown 1996). In a Hungarian study, Tamas *et al.* (1996) reported that insulin requirements increased by up to 3 units per day in the premenstrual phase of the cycle. If ignored or left untreated this could cause an increased risk of women developing DKA on a monthly basis.

8. Emotional stress

Emotional stress appears to have unpredictable effects on a person's blood glucose level. Indeed, many people who are newly diagnosed with diabetes often complain that they have had a very stressful year emotionally and have then developed diabetes as well.

9. Drugs

Certain drugs have been found to contribute to the development of hyperglycaemia and potentially to DKA. These include steroids, thiazide diuretics and tricyclic antidepressants. Therefore, when these drugs are prescribed their potential effects on blood glucose levels need to be monitored and treatment adjusted accordingly.

Treatment and management of DKA

Treatment should commence immediately the person's vital signs relating to airway, breathing and circulation have been assessed and are stable. Management should be based upon individual assessment, reassessment and need.

1. Treatment
Treatment in relation to DKA is three-fold.

To correct the fluid and electrolyte disturbances
Intravenous access will be required, therefore if peripheral access proves difficult, it may be necessary to insert a central line. Fluid replacement should begin immediately and should be rapid initially, with the aim of replacing approximately 6 litres of fluid within the first 24 hours (Levy 2006).

The rate of fluid replacement has been a cause for concern over recent years with large volumes being associated with the risk of cerebral oedema, particularly in children, and carrying a high mortality rate of 21–24%, with 15–26% of survivors left with permanent neurological injury (Sharma *et al.* 2007).

Sodium chloride (0.9%) should be given intravenously to begin with, but as the blood glucose levels fall to below 15 mmol/l this should be changed to 5% dextrose. If the blood glucose rises to above 15 mmol/l with the introduction of the dextrose infusion, it is not recommended that the infusion is changed back to sodium chloride. Instead, the amount of insulin being given at the same time should be increased (Savage and Kilvert 2006).

To raise intracellular and lower extracellular levels of glucose
Insulin   Neither sodium chloride nor glucose infusions should be given alone and low-dose intravenous insulin therapy should accompany the fluid replacement. The main action of insulin when used in DKA is to prevent gluconeogenesis by the liver and worsening of the condition. Low-dose insulin regimens (5–10 units/hour) have been found to be as effective as high-dose regimens ranging from 50 to 100 units/hour in reducing blood glucose levels but, in addition, low-dose regimens had the added benefit of reducing the risk of hypokalaemia and hypoglycaemia (Henriksen *et al.* 2006).

Intravenous variable-dose insulin is given in these circumstances via a sliding-scale regimen. A schedule of how many units of insulin should be given per hour is drawn up, based on the calculation of 0.1 unit/kg/hour (Diabetes UK 2001). The amount given each hour is dependent on the person's current blood glucose level. The number of units prescribed should also take into account people who are insulin resistant and/or septic, as they may need more units of insulin per kilogram of body weight per hour (Savage and Kilvert 2006). Therefore, as the person's blood glucose level drops the amount of insulin given per hour will be reduced accordingly.

As the blood glucose level falls, the insulin infusion can be reduced to 0.05 units/kg/hour and should be continued until the patient is clinically stable and has resumed eating and drinking.

Key point

When treating a person with a sliding-scale insulin regimen, the person's blood glucose level should never be allowed to drop below 4 mmol/l as this will initiate compensatory mechanisms by the body associated with hypoglycaemia. The resultant low blood glucose levels can also be very distressing for the patient.

Potassium As all patients presenting with DKA will be potassium depleted, this will require careful monitoring and the addition of 20 mmol of potassium with every 500 ml of intravenous fluid. This can be discontinued once the ketoacidosis has resolved and blood potassium levels are within the normal parameters.

Sodium Patients may have low sodium levels but these are compensated for in the saline infusion and tend to return to within normal limits as the blood glucose level falls. Therefore, it is generally not necessary to give extra sodium.

To increase the blood pH
The administration of insulin is usually sufficient to increase the blood pH level; however, if the acidosis is slow to resolve and the blood glucose is <10 mmol/l it may be beneficial to change the 5% glucose infusion to a 10% glucose infusion (Savage and Kilvert 2006). This allows for a higher rate of insulin to be given, which will exert a greater effect on raising blood pH.

Bicarbonate administration has been associated with the development of cerebral oedema and hypokalaemia (Williams and Pickup 2004) and is therefore avoided as a treatment modality in DKA. However, it may become necessary if the patient is not responding to rehydration and insulin therapy and their blood pH value remains <7.0. If bicarbonate is prescribed, the patient needs to be managed in a high dependency/intensive care unit and monitored carefully for signs of cerebral oedema and cardiac arrhythmias.

2. Management
Savage and Kilvert (2006) recommend that laboratory blood glucose levels should be measured at diagnosis and every 2 hours thereafter. Capillary blood glucose measurements via a hand-held meter should also be recorded hourly until they are stable and within normal limits.

Urea, electrolytes and bicarbonate levels should be checked 2 hours following admission and then 4-hourly until the patient's condition is stable and the bicarbonate level is above 15 mmol/l.

Neurological status should be assessed hourly and an hourly record of fluid input and output should be maintained to observe for renal function and circulatory overload. It would also be prudent to attach the patient to a cardiac monitor and observe for any T-wave changes, which may be an indication of hypokalaemia (Diabetes UK 2001).

In Pippa's case, she would be cared for in a high dependency/intensive care unit due to the high level of monitoring and observation that is required. All of the above management recommendations would be implemented and reassurances given to both Pippa and her parents. Once she starts to feel better, and the diabetic ketoacidosis abates, Pippa can begin eating and drinking and can be transferred on to a subcutaneous insulin regimen.

Key point

It should be noted that urinary ketones often take some time to clear but this should not delay the commencement or return to subcutaneous insulin.

The process of ascertaining the reason for the onset of DKA should then begin so that the patient can be helped to prevent a further occurrence. In Pippa's case, she will require education and support on all aspects relating to diabetes and its treatment to enable her to self-manage the condition.

Hypoglycaemia

Definition

Hypoglycaemia is a serious, frightening, potentially debilitating and fatal complication of both type 1 and type 2 diabetes. As a result many people with diabetes will never achieve optimum glycaemic control as the fear of hypoglycaemia is so great that they prefer to maintain their blood glucose levels higher than necessary 'just to be on the safe side'.

The occurrence of hypoglycaemia in those with type 2 diabetes and in the elderly has been associated with serious morbidity, including a significant increase in the risk of stroke, myocardial infarction, acute cardiac failure and ventricular arrhythmias (Zammitt and Frier 2005).

The problem of hypoglycaemia has been recognized since the introduction of insulin in 1922 but it has increased in frequency, particularly with the publication of the Diabetes Control and Complications Trial (1997). This large, 10-year study concluded that intensive glycaemic therapy was the key to significantly reducing the development of the long-term complications of diabetes. Within the study, the lowest incidence of complications was found among people who achieved blood glucose levels averaging 8.6 mmol/l and had HbA1c levels of around 7%. The downside of these findings is that as patients and healthcare practitioners strive to achieve these results, treatment is intensified and the margin of blood glucose error becomes smaller, thus increasing the incidence of hypoglycaemia.

Hypoglycaemia is not just a side-effect of insulin; it can also occur in people taking oral antidiabetes agents that act by increasing the production of endogenous insulin, such as sulphonylureas and prandial glucose regulators. This specific side-effect is often overlooked by patients and healthcare professionals and many people with type 2 diabetes have little knowledge of the symptoms and treatment of hypoglycaemia (Thomson *et al.* 1991).

Hypoglycaemia is defined as a blood glucose level ≤3.9 mmol/l (American Diabetes Association 2005a) but Diabetes UK use the slogan 'Four is the Floor' working on the principle that blood glucose levels should not fall below 4.0 mmol/l. The figure of 3.9 mmol/l has been derived from studies that have shown that this is the level at which the normal glucose counter-regulatory system to raise falling blood glucose levels is triggered in people who do not have diabetes (Mitrakou *et al.* 1991; Fanelli 1994). However, the definition of hypoglycaemia needs to be extended to include any episode of an abnormally low plasma glucose concentration that exposes the individual to potential harm (American Diabetes Association 2005a).

Debates have ensued about whether episodes of hypoglycaemia can be accurately reported when the person has relied solely upon the warning signs and symptoms and a blood glucose has not been recorded at the time. It is accepted that people with diabetes learn to recognize signs of impending and actual hypoglycaemia and treat them accordingly, but there may be times when co-morbid conditions or therapies may produce similar symptoms to those of hypoglycaemia. In order to rule out the presence of other factors, it is important for people to measure their blood glucose levels when they suspect they are experiencing hypoglycaemia.

Pathophysiology of hypoglycaemia

In order to function normally, the human brain requires a constant supply of glucose via the blood stream as it is unable to synthesize or store glucose and therefore, by default, is extremely sensitive to glucose deprivation. To protect the integrity of the brain and ultimately the life of the person, several physiological mechanisms have evolved to respond to, and limit, the deleterious effects of hypoglycaemia.

In the event of hypoglycaemia, three main neuroendocrine counter-regulatory responses are activated simultaneously:

1. The alpha cells in the Islets of Langerhans detect falling blood glucose levels and respond by suppressing the release of insulin and increasing the release of glucagon. The increased levels of glucagon are transported to the liver where they stimulate the release of stored glucose via glycogenolysis and the production of glucose through the process of gluconeogenesis.
2. The presence of hypoglycaemia is also recognized by the hypothalamic glucose sensor in the brain, which responds by activating the sympathetic nervous

system to release adrenaline. This in turn increases glucose synthesis and release by the liver, thus increasing blood glucose levels. Within the counter-regulatory mechanism, the action of glucagon and adrenaline are the principle defences (Page and Hall 1999).

3. At the same time as the above, the anterior pituitary gland secretes adreno-corticotrophic hormone (ACTH), which in turn causes the adrenal glands to release cortisol. Cortisol has the same effect on the liver as glucagon in that it increases gluconeogenesis and glycogenolysis, resulting in increased blood glucose levels. Growth hormone is also released by the anterior pituitary gland, which influences hepatic glucose release. However, cortisol and growth hormone also reduce the amount of glucose that is deposited in the peripheral tissues, but this effect takes several hours to become manifest. As a result, it is thought that cortisol and growth hormone do not have a significant role to play in the acute hypoglycaemic phase, but are important hormones in prolonged hypoglycaemia.

Hypoglycaemic unawareness

In some people with diabetes, the normal pathophysiology of the glucose counter-regulatory mechanism becomes impaired. This tends to be the result of repeated hypoglycaemic episodes in which the normal glucose counter-regulatory mechanism is activated to raise blood glucose levels but is unable to do so because insulin levels do not decrease; once insulin has been injected it cannot then be withdrawn and will continue to act accordingly – glucagon levels do not increase and the increase in adrenaline levels is weakened. It is this attenuated adrenal response that causes the clinical syndrome of 'hypoglycaemic unawareness' (American Diabetes Association 2005a). In hypoglycaemic unawareness, the warning signs that previously allowed the person to recognize hypoglycaemia developing and take appropriate action to treat it are lost. This can result in a person compromising their own personal safety and the safety of others in the event of a hypoglycaemic episode.

Hypoglycaemia awareness can be regained with an intensive training programme, which requires regular blood glucose testing and regular snacks between meals to avoid hypoglycaemia at all costs. Once the glucose counter-regulatory response has been 'reset' hypoglycaemic warning signs should return and the person can then aim to gradually reduce their blood glucose levels.

Case study: Jerry

Jerry has been brought into the local Accident and Emergency unit today as he was found by his wife slumped on the kitchen floor, semi-conscious and not able to respond to her questions or commands. He is 74 years of age and

Continued

it generally very fit and active; however, over the past few weeks he has been complaining of feeling 'wobbly and shaky' and hungry, mainly in a morning before breakfast. His wife has commented that sometimes first thing in a morning Jerry can be obstructive and awkward, which is out of character. Once he has had breakfast he feels better and the symptoms disappear. These changes in character and malaise do not occur every day, but on average one to two times per week.

He has recently gained approximately 10 kg in weight, which he is now very motivated to lose. For the past 6 weeks he has been following a diet plan given to him by the hospital dietitian, which has enabled him to reduce his weight by 3 kg. He is very pleased with his weight loss to date, but would like the weekly loss to be greater so that he is able to achieve his goal weight sooner. He would also like to improve his overall physical fitness as he has not been doing any form of regular exercise for the past 5 years. He has therefore joined an elderly person's swimming club and now swims for 45 minutes one to two times per week in the evening.

Past medical history

- Type 2 diabetes for the past 11 years.
- Hypertension.
- Hyperlipidaemia.
- He has recently developed background retinopathy and a small neuropathic foot ulcer on the little toe of his left foot as a result of his diabetes.

Family history

- Married to Gladys for the past 49 years.
- Has two grown-up sons in their 30s but they live a distance away from Jerry and Gladys. Both are fit and well and do not have diabetes.
- Mother died of a stroke secondary to type 2 diabetes at the age of 72 years.
- Father died of an acute myocardial infarction aged 59 years.

Medication

- Glibenclamide 10 mg daily, split into two equal doses taken with his breakfast and evening meal.
- Metformin 2 g per day split into 2 equal doses and taken with breakfast and evening meal.
- Simvastatin 10 mg once daily.
- Losartan 50 mg once daily.

Allergies

- Elastoplast®.

Examination

- Semi-conscious, able to open eyes to verbal commands. Not responding verbally.
- Poor co-ordination.
- Temperature   36.8°C.
- Pulse   121 bpm, regular.
- Blood pressure   160/85 mmHg.
- Venous blood glucose   6.4 mmol/l.
- HbA1c   9.2%.
- Urinalysis – negative to ketones, glucose, protein and blood.
- Body mass index (BMI)   31 kg/m^2.
- Waist circumference   125 cm.

Discussion of Jerry's case

Careful assessment and thought needs to be given to unravel the case that Jerry presents, as his presenting signs and symptoms are not as obvious as they might be.

In considering his lifestyle, over time he has gained a significant amount of weight and his BMI is within the obese category. As a consequence, he will have a decreased level of insulin sensitivity, requiring increasing amounts of anti-diabetes medication. However, now that he is losing weight effectively and is exercising regularly this trend can be reversed and his insulin sensitivity can be increased, which would require a reduction in his antidiabetes medication. If his medication is not reviewed and potentially reduced, he will be at an increased risk of hypoglycaemia.

Signs and symptoms

The risk of hypoglycaemia in a person with diabetes is highest before meals and during the night. In the case study, Jerry is complaining of feeling 'wobbly and shaky' and hungry in a morning and his wife has noticed him being obstructive and awkward. These are classic signs of hypoglycaemia. Feelings of hunger and instability occur as a direct result of the sympathetic nervous system being activated and increased amounts of adrenaline being released. In more severe, untreated cases of hypoglycaemia, the person develops neuroglycopaenic symptoms, which include confusion, behaviour that is out of character, inability to concentrate, drowsiness, visual disturbances and tingling of the mouth and lips. On 2–3 days of the week, Jerry appears to be exhibiting neuroglycopaenic symptoms.

In trying to unpick and problem solve the information in the case study, it is concluded that in losing weight Jerry has increased his insulin sensitivity, thus the endogenous insulin that he is producing is working more effectively, thereby reducing the amount of endogenous insulin he needs to produce to maintain glycaemic homeostasis. As the dose of his glibenclamide, which is a long-acting sulphonylurea, has not been reduced, insulin continues to be secreted in amounts excessive to his need. In addition, his metformin will continue to decrease insulin resistance and make the circulating insulin even more effective. It appears that Jerry has a low blood glucose level some mornings, which he is treating unknowingly by having his breakfast. It is for these reasons that glibenclamide is no longer a drug of choice in treating type 2 diabetes and practitioners are now opting for shorter-acting sulphonylureas, such as glipizide and gliclazide, to reduce the risk of hypoglycaemia.

The mornings in which Jerry shows neuroglycopaenic symptoms of hypoglycaemia by his obstructive and awkward behaviour are most likely to be on the days after he has been swimming the night before. The action of exercise reduces blood glucose levels and will therefore worsen any potential hypoglycaemic episodes if left untreated.

Diagnosing hypoglycaemia

Jerry does not present a typical case as his venous blood glucose level is technically within the normal parameter of 4–7 mmol/l; however, his high HbA1c indicates that his diabetes control is poor and his blood glucose levels are probably regularly above 12 mmol/l. As mentioned previously, hypoglycaemia is technically defined as a blood glucose level of <4 mmol/l.

In people who regularly have high blood glucose levels their glucose counter-regulatory system can become defective and 'reset' itself so that it becomes activated at a higher blood glucose level. This is what has happened in Jerry's case and can be corrected by gradually over time, reducing the high blood glucose levels so that they fall within normal limits.

While the urinalysis reading in Jerry's case cannot confirm hypoglycaemia, it supports the diagnosis by the absence of ketones and glucose.

As Jerry is not being treated with insulin, he has not made the connection between oral antidiabetes medication and the development of hypoglycaemia. Jerry and his wife will need to be educated on the causes and treatment of hypoglycaemia and the importance of measuring blood glucose levels when hypoglycaemia is suspected. This will aid a clearer diagnosis and rule out the presence of other co-morbidities, which may cause similar symptoms

Causes of hypoglycaemia

The main causes of hypoglycaemia are: (1) the result of having injected or stimulated the endogenous release of too much active insulin; or (2) there is not enough circulating glucose for the amount of insulin taken or released. This can occur in the following circumstances.

1. Excessive doses of insulin

This can occur if the person has miscalculated or misdialled on the insulin pen too many insulin units to meet their body requirements, or if they have been prescribed or are taking too much oral antidiabetes medication that stimulates their own production of insulin, as is the case with sulphonylureas and prandial glucose regulators. In these circumstances, the active circulating insulin requires sufficient amounts of glucose to act upon and prevent hypoglycaemia.

2. Absorption rate of insulin

While the correct amount of insulin may have been injected, an erratic or unpredictable absorption rate can contribute to the development of hypoglycaemia. It is anticipated that once insulin is injected it will perform to its expected profile; however, different situations may alter its absorption rate. Absorption rates tend to differ depending on where the injection has been given. The abdomen has the highest absorption rate, with the arms being slightly slower and the thigh slower still. Therefore if someone is used to injecting into their thigh each morning, changing to injecting into the abdomen, which has a higher absorption rate, could lead to hypoglycaemia.

Additionally, a rise in skin temperature will cause vasodilation and an increase in insulin absorption, making hypoglycaemia particularly prevalent after a hot bath or sauna. Inadvertent intramuscular rather than subcutaneous injection of insulin will also create a more rapid absorption of insulin.

The presence of lipohypertrophy may affect the absorption of insulin. These are fatty lumps that develop as a consequence of repeatedly using the same insulin injection site. They are caused by the effect of insulin stimulating the growth of fat tissue and if injected into lead to an erratic absorption of insulin. In this instance, no insulin may be delivered initially, followed by copious amounts of insulin being later released that does not correspond with rising blood glucose levels.

3. Delayed or missed meals

Once insulin has been injected, or the production of endogenous insulin has been stimulated via oral medication, this will continue to be active, whether or not the person has eaten. It is therefore vitally important to ensure that the action of insulin and medication is understood and taken appropriately and in conjunction with food. The rising action of insulin needs to be given or stimulated so that it closely matches the rising blood glucose levels when the person eats if hypoglycaemia is to be avoided.

4. Exercise

Exercise will increase the rate at which insulin is absorbed by the subcutaneous tissues and therefore the normal action of insulin becomes more effective.

5. Malabsorption

This relates to malabsorption of glucose, rather than malabsorption of insulin. People with type 1 diabetes are more susceptible to developing coeliac disease, which results in an unpredictable absorption of glucose in the small intestine. This makes matching insulin requirements to rising blood glucose levels very difficult and increases the risk of hypoglycaemia.

6. Alcohol

In patients with diabetes treated with insulin, alcohol has been found to account for up to one-fifth of hospital attendances for hypoglycaemia (Potter *et al.* 1982, cited in Richardson *et al.* 2005). Few studies have been conducted on the effect of alcohol on blood glucose levels but it has been associated with hypoglycaemia in a variety of ways. First, ingestion of even small amounts of alcohol can impair the person's ability to detect an impending hypoglycaemic event and therefore make them less likely to take evasive action. Second, some studies have shown a relationship between alcohol ingestion and an impaired glucose counter-regulatory response in which hepatic gluconeogenesis and glycogenolysis is reduced, making recovery from hypoglycaemia more prolonged and difficult.

A study by Richardson *et al.* (2005) confirmed that modest amounts of alcohol taken with an evening meal positively correlated with an increased risk of delayed hypoglycaemia, which mainly occurred the following morning in patients with type 1 diabetes. This emphasizes the need to educate patients on the effects of alcohol on blood glucose levels in attempts to reduce their risk of experiencing a hypoglycaemic episode.

Treatment and management

1. Initial treatment

The aim of treatment for hypoglycaemia is to restore the blood glucose levels back to within normal limits for the individual as quickly as possible.

Key point

As a rule of thumb, 15 g of fast-acting carbohydrate will increase a person's blood glucose level by 2 mmol/l within 20 minutes.

Conscious, co-operative patient

In the conscious person this can be done quickly and easily by making sure that they have continuous access to fast-acting carbohydrates, such as glucose. The following items contain 10–15 g of carbohydrate, which may be suitable for treating hypoglycaemia in a conscious, co-operative patient:

- Two to three 5 g glucose tablets.
- 120–175 ml orange juice.

- A handful of raisins.
- Half a can of a cola or other soft drink – not diet.
- 6–10 jellybeans or gumdrops.
- 2 teaspoons or cubes of sugar.
- 2 teaspoons of honey.
- Glucose paste (GlucoGel®). This is a 40% dextrose gel, which is supplied in a squeezable 25 g tube or a single 80 g bottle. Each tube of GlucoGel® contains a measure of 10 g carbohydrate, and each bottle contains 32 g carbohydrate. It is administered by squeezing the gel into the mouth and the person swallowing it. Alternatively, GlucoGel® can be squeezed inside the cheek, and the outside of the cheek gently rubbed to aid absorption.
- 175–235 ml of non-fat or 1% milk. Non-fat milk is specifically mentioned.

Key point

The fats found in milk and chocolate, which are commonly taken by patients when they perceive their blood glucose level to be low, should be avoided as they delay the absorption of the glucose and therefore slow down the recovery rate from the hypoglycaemic episode.

If the blood glucose level is particularly low then the above amounts may need to be doubled to give a rise of 4 mmol/l. The person's blood glucose level should be tested 10–15 minutes after treatment has been initiated and the process repeated if the blood glucose level remains low.

Uncooperative, semi/unconscious patient
Giving oral glucose to an uncooperative or semi/unconscious patient is clearly dangerous and could cause them to choke to death. Therefore other solutions are available and should be accessible for the person with diabetes.

Glucagon   Glucagon increases blood glucose by stimulating glycogen breakdown in the liver and is supplied as a powder in a vial with a needle, syringe and diluant. It works most rapidly when given intravenously but, if this is not convenient or possible, it can also be given intramuscularly or subcutaneously. When given it should restore consciousness in patients within approximately 10 minutes (Page and Hall 1999). Glucagon will be relatively ineffective in people who are thin, malnourished, starving, anorexic or alcoholic, as they are prone to poor hepatic glycogen stores (Levy 2006).

Intravenous dextrose   Intravenous dextrose, if available, remains the most rapid and effective treatment for a severe hypoglycaemic attack. It is recommended as a first-line treatment in most Accident and Emergency departments and is particularly useful if glucagon has already been given but has not been effective.

A 50 ml dose of 50% dextrose will increase a person's blood glucose level approximately 12.5 mmol/l within 5 minutes of administration. As the solution is viscous it should be given into an antecubital vein to minimize the risk of thrombophlebitis and thrombosis (Levy 2006).

2. Follow-up treatment (all patients)

By administering a fast-acting, simple carbohydrate the person's blood glucose level will rise quickly making them feel much better within a few minutes. However, to avoid the blood glucose level plummeting again as quickly as it rose, it is vital that the initial treatment is followed up by giving the patient a longer-acting, complex carbohydrate.

If at the time of the hypoglycaemic episode the person was about to eat a meal, they should be positively encouraged to do this. If the hypoglycaemia occurs between meals the person should be given a sandwich; or two or three biscuits that contain oats to offer a slower absorption of the sugars; or a bowl of cereal that has a low glycaemic index.

Ascertaining the cause of the hypoglycaemia and educating the person and their significant others on the causes and treatment of low blood glucose levels are the crucial next steps in helping to prevent or reduce the occurrence of hypoglycaemic events.

Conclusion

The two main diabetes emergencies, hyperglycaemia and hypoglycaemia, have been highlighted and discussed in this chapter. For each of these conditions the relevant pathophysiology has been described to provide an understanding of what happens in the body when the blood glucose levels become raised or fall below the normal parameters. The main causes of high and low blood glucose levels have been considered and the immediate and acute management of each of the conditions identified.

Through the use of the two case studies and the discussion of these, readers have been encouraged to problem solve some of the not so obvious issues that patients with hyperglycaemia or hypoglycaemia may present with. As hyperglycaemia and hypoglycaemia are both life-threatening conditions, it is hoped that this chapter will help to ensure that a correct and prompt diagnosis is made and the most appropriate treatment administered without delay. Emphasis then needs to be given to understanding the cause of the abnormal blood glucose level and taking steps to avoid repeat performances.

4

Diabetes in the medical ward

Aims of the chapter

This chapter will:

1. Identify and discuss the different types of neuropathy, including the peripheral neuropathies and autonomic neuropathy.
2. Discuss factors that can contribute to the onset of neuropathy developing in a person with diabetes.
3. Critically problem solve the short- and long-term management and education of a person with neuropathy that has led to the development of a neuropathic foot ulcer requiring hospitalization.

Diabetes is the most common cause of foot problems and non-traumatic leg amputation, both of which place a significant demand on National Health Service resources and monies in the UK. It has been calculated that 7% of people with diabetes in westernized countries have a foot ulcer at any given time and diabetic foot problems account for 20% of the total costs allocated from the National Health Service budget for diabetes care (Williams and Pickup 2004).

This chapter details the care of a patient with diabetes admitted to a medical ward with a neuropathic foot ulcer. The different types of neuropathy that develop as a complication of diabetes are discussed and the potential causes of neuropathy are highlighted. Strategies relating to the improvement of diabetes control that can subsequently reduce the incidence of neuropathy are given.

Diabetic neuropathy

Neuropathy is one of the more common microvascular complications that can arise as a consequence of having diabetes and long-term, suboptimal blood glucose control. People with diabetes have a 30–50% risk over their lifetime of developing chronic peripheral neuropathy, and 10–20% of these will go on to develop severe neuropathic symptoms (Marshall and Flyvbjerg 2006). While diabetic neuropathy encompasses a number of different neuropathic syndromes including focal, multifocal and autonomic neuropathy, all of which will be considered in this chapter, by far the most common form of neuropathy is distal symmetrical sensory polyneuropathy (DSP) (Tesfaye and Kempler 2005).

Distal symmetrical sensory polyneuropathy (DSP)

DSP has been defined as 'the presence of symptoms and/or signs of peripheral nerve dysfunction in people with diabetes after the exclusion of other causes' (Boulton *et al.* 1998). The two main clinical consequences of DSP are foot ulceration, sometimes culminating in painful neuropathy, and limb amputation, both of which are associated with high rates of patient morbidity and mortality (Boulton *et al.* 2004).

DSP occurs as a result of prolonged high blood glucose levels leading to intracellular hyperglycaemia. This stimulates a complex biochemical process, culminating in microvascular changes. As a result of these microvascular changes, endoneural hypoxia develops causing small and large nerve fibre dysfunction (Levy 2006). Intracellular hyperglycaemia also causes activation of growth factors, which results in endothelial and connective tissue damage. These are discussed in more detail in Chapter 6.

Charcot neuroarthropathy

Charcot neuropathy is an acute, destructive disease process of the foot causing significant bone and foot joint destruction, leading to profound foot deformity (Figure 4.1). Fortunately, it is an uncommon complication of neuropathy but is characteristically seen in patients with long-standing type 1 diabetes who have other advanced microvascular complications, such as retinopathy requiring laser treatment and nephropathy (Levy 2006). It can also occur in those with type 2 diabetes, but this is less typical. It is caused by an increased blood flow to the foot, which predisposes to a thinning of the bones of the feet as the minerals in the foot are simply 'washed away', leading to a condition called diabetic osteopaenia.

Charcot neuropathy usually presents as an acute onset in which there is a history of a minor injury to the foot that may have gone unnoticed for some time. On inspection, there is a unilateral erythema with accompanying oedema and the affected foot is at least 2°C hotter than the non-affected foot. This is measured with an infra-red thermometer and at this point it is important to determine if the swelling is due to cellulitis or Charcot neuroarthropathy. Generally, cellulitis is more common with neuropathic foot ulcers that have become infected.

About a third of patients complain of pain or discomfort at this time, but if an X-ray were taken it is highly likely that it would be unremarkable and the bones of the foot would be presented as 'normal'. However, a bone scan done at the same time would indicate early evidence of bone destruction. If left untreated

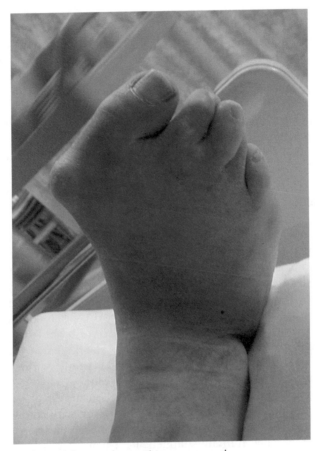

Figure 4.1   Gross bone deformity due to Charcot neuropathy.

and the condition progresses, over a period of just a few weeks the patient may begin to notice the shape of their foot changing and they may experience an alteration in the sensation of the foot or experience the sound of bones crunching when they walk. The affected foot typically develops a 'rocker bottom' appearance, which causes hot spots for the development of pressure ulcers on the plantar aspects. There will be evidence of new bone formation, and partial and complete dislocation of the joints.

Early diagnosis is essential and if 'in doubt' always treat for Charcot foot initially, until a firm diagnosis is made. The aim of treatment is complete immobilization until such a time as there is no longer any X-ray evidence of the bone destruction continuing and the temperature of the affected foot is within 2°C of the contralateral foot. Remobilization needs to be undertaken very gradually to prevent further bone destruction.

Autonomic neuropathy

Along with DSP, autonomic neuropathy is a common condition in people with diabetes and results from damage to the sympathetic and parasympathetic nerves. It is a serious condition that should not be treated lightly as it can affect a number of systems in the body, causing significant morbidity and leading to mortality.

As autonomic neuropathy can cause damage and disruption to different parts of the body, the clinical signs and symptoms are varied and diverse but tend to be linked mainly to the cardiovascular, gastrointestinal and genitourinary systems.

1. Cardiovascular autonomic neuropathy

Cardiovascular autonomic neuropathy receives a great deal of attention in patients with diabetes due to the high levels of mortality associated with it. A resting tachycardia and postural hypotension without an appropriate heart rate response may indicate damage to the cardiovascular nervous system. In these cases, people are more at risk of experiencing a 'silent' myocardial infarction (MI) where the patient does not experience the characteristic stabbing chest pain during cardiac infarction due to the neuropathic nerve damage. MI is often not detected until a later date when an electrocardiogram is performed for other reasons.

People with neuropathy affecting the cardiovascular system are also at a greatly increased risk of sudden death. Indeed, 80% of all people with type 2 diabetes will die prematurely of a cardiovascular-related event.

While it is generally accepted that regular exercise can help to reduce hypertension in the general population, this differs in the person with autonomic neuropathy. In these people, hypotension or hypertension can develop after vigorous exercise, especially when initially commencing a new exercise regimen. In addition, these people have difficulty in controlling their body temperature, which can have implications for the person if they exercise in hot or cold environments (Boulton *et al.* 2005).

2. Gastrointestinal autonomic neuropathy

Autonomic neuropathy can cause gastrointestinal disturbances, including gastroparesis. This should be suspected in individuals who have unexplained erratic blood glucose control, as it may be due to delayed emptying of the stomach contents. If the cause of this is found to be gastroparesis then glycaemic control can often be restored in these people, initially by delaying diabetes treatment, including insulin, until after the patient has eaten. Constipation alternating with episodes of diarrhoea is another common symptom of gastrointestinal autonomic neuropathy and an endoscopy may be required to rule out other potential causes. Furthermore, patients with autonomic neuropathy affecting the gastrointestinal tract may complain of gustatory sweating, where they perspire profusely on the forehead, face, scalp and neck after eating a meal. Individuals comment that this is an uncomfortable and embarrassing symptom of the condition.

3. Genitourinary autonomic neuropathy

The genitourinary tract is also affected by autonomic neuropathy, leading to disturbances of the bladder and/or sexual organs. This should be suspected if the individual experiences recurrent urinary tract infections, pyelonephritis, urinary retention or incontinence, which arises due to poor-quality nerve impulses and control in the affected organs. It can also cause loss of penile erection and/or retrograde ejaculation in men. In these cases a full medical, sexual and psychological history should be taken to exclude other potential causes.

Focal and multifocal neuropathies

Mono or focal neuropathies may have a sudden onset and typically involve one specific nerve. They occur most frequently in older patients with type 2 diabetes. The most common nerves affected are the median, ulnar and common peroneal nerves, which become trapped requiring decompression or develop demyelination and axonal degeneration. While it is extremely rare, the cranial nerves III, IV, VI and VII have also been known to be at risk of neuropathic damage, thought to develop as a result of a microvascular infarct. Fortunately, this usually resolves itself spontaneously over a period of months (Boulton *et al.* 2005).

Uni- or bilateral muscle weakness and wasting of the proximal thigh muscles can also develop in this type of neuropathy, potentially causing gait and mobility difficulties.

Peripheral vascular disease

Peripheral vascular disease associated with diabetes is defined as the presence of an abnormal narrowing or occlusion, usually due to atheroscleroma in the main arteries, including the arteries of the lower limbs, giving rise to ischaemia in the feet. When peripheral vascular disease is combined with diabetes, a marked increase in mortality rate and risk of limb amputation is noted (Bloomgarden 2007). The general presence of atheroscleroma renders the person with diabetes at a two to five times increased risk of coronary and cerebrovascular disease when compared to the general population (Marshall and Flyvbjerg 2006). Additionally, people with diabetes have an average reduction in life expectancy of 5–10 years, predominantly due to premature cardiovascular disease.

In approximately half of the patients who develop peripheral vascular disease, no symptoms are experienced; approximately 15% develop claudication; and 33% report difficulty in walking. The remaining 1–2% have critical limb ischaemia with pain on rest, and an increased likelihood of developing foot ulcers or gangrene (Bloomgarden 2007).

The strongest risk factors for peripheral vascular disease include smoking, hypertension, hyperlipidaemia and albuminuria (Marshall and Flyvbjerg 2006), all of which need to be regularly assessed and actively addressed to help prevent the development of such potentially devastating diabetes-related complications.

These risk factors and their prevention and treatment are discussed in greater detail in Chapter 6.

Peripheral vascular disease of the foot

Peripheral vascular disease of the foot can present in different ways. Severe peripheral vascular disease can cause the foot to become pink and painful, with the absence of any pedal pulses. This state indicates that ulceration may be imminent. Alternatively, a sudden occlusion of the popliteal or superficial femoral artery will result in a pale, painful foot that is cold to touch and has a purple, mottled effect. In this instance, the person is at high risk of developing necrosis of the toes (Edmonds and Foster 2000).

Measurement of the ankle–brachial index is one test that is used to confirm peripheral vascular disease but is not found to be a reliable indicator in people who also have diabetes. This is because it is very difficult to adequately compress the blood vessels during the test, thus giving rise to inaccurate, unhelpful readings. Other methods that may aid diagnosis include the use of magnetic resonance scans and computerized tomography angiography if available.

As a precautionary measure, people with diabetes and peripheral vascular disease should be advised to have their toe nails cut and any callus removed by a trained podiatrist, as any accidental injury to their foot can lead to ulceration and potential amputation. It is for these reasons that 'over the counter' callus/veruccae removal preparations should also be avoided.

Screening and diagnosing diabetic neuropathy

Given the potentially devastating effects of diabetic neuropathy and the fact that many of the symptoms are potentially treatable, it is important to screen all patients with diabetes on a regular basis, at least annually. In addition, prompt identification and intervention may prevent or delay the progression of the disease, thus reducing patient morbidity and mortality.

The presence of DSP is specifically assessed by carefully examining the person's feet for any areas of pressure, ulceration or shape abnormality. Autonomic nerve damage leads to reduced sweating, resulting in dry and cracked areas of the skin, which make the person susceptible to infection (Williams and Pickup 2004). Areas around the foot and lower limb can be assessed for the presence of DSP by the use of a 10 g monofilament, which is a standard, properly calibrated device.

Without the patient seeing, the monofilament should be applied perpendicular to the skin surface on at least five different points on the sole of the foot (Figure 4.2). Sufficient force should then be applied to the filament to cause it to bend or buckle. The patient should be asked to indicate when they are able to feel the pressure applied and in which foot the pressure is felt. During the process, the filament should not be in contact with the skin at each testing site for longer than 2 seconds. Decreased sensation at any of the sites tested has been shown to produce an 18-fold increase in the risk of the patient developing a neuropathic ulcer (McNeely et al. 1995).

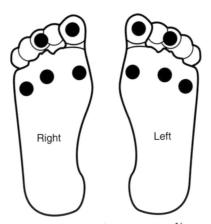

Figure 4.2 Areas of the foot to be tested with a 10 g monofilament.

Vibration perception threshold is another method used to screen for neuropathy. It has been shown that an inability to feel the vibrating head of a neurothesiometer at >25 V when placed on the padded area of the big toe is an indication that the person is at high risk of developing a neuropathic foot ulcer.

Screening should also include taking a comprehensive and accurate history from the patient, specifically asking them about the effect of vigorous exercise, the presence of chest pain and their ability to control their body temperature. Questions should also centre around their gastrointestinal function and whether they have experienced any changes in this, including the presence of gustatory sweating. Assessment of the person's genitourinary tract should also be included, in which doors can be opened to give people the opportunity to discuss any sensitive, sexual concerns they may have.

Treatment of neuropathic foot ulcers

The adage 'prevention is better than cure' is certainly applicable to the screening and treatment of neuropathic foot ulcers. Good glycaemic control, where the person consistently achieves a haemoglobin A1c (HbA1c) level of between 6.5 and 7.5% is paramount in halting or delaying the disease process.

Glycaemic control

The Diabetes Control and Complications Trial (1997) found that for those people who had their diabetes treated intensively and were able to maintain their blood glucose levels within the target range, the appearance of neuropathy was reduced by 69% in the primary prevention group. This group was classified as those patients who had no signs of retinopathy at the start of the trial and achieved an average blood glucose level of 8.6 mmol/l with an HbA1c level of around 7%.

For those people who at the start of the trial had signs of eye disease but had their diabetes treated as intensively as the primary control group, the risk of developing further neuropathy was reduced by 57%. Both are very significant results, particularly when applied to the potential reduction in mortality and improved quality of life for a large number of people with diabetes.

Patient education

Patient education surrounding the importance of foot health and the potential complications needs to be instigated at the time of diagnosing diabetes. All people with diabetes should be informed regularly of the need to carefully inspect their feet on a daily basis. In the presence of neuropathy, it is possible for the person to step on a sharp object and not feel any pain, causing the object to become embedded in the foot and causing untold complications. In addition, walking barefoot should be discouraged at all times and patients advised to regularly sweep and vacuum the floors of their houses. Also, something as simple as new shoes can cause rubbing and blisters that may go undetected due to the lack of any pain sensation, but have the potential of developing into deleterious foot ulcers.

When inspecting each foot the person should consider the colour of the skin and determine whether it looks pink and well perfused. Any signs of a deformity or swelling should be observed for, also whether there is any evidence of callus formation or breakdown in the skin. If lesions are present on the foot, these should be assessed for signs of infection or necrosis.

People who are not flexible or mobile enough to carefully inspect the soles of their feet can be encouraged to use a mirror to perform this task. Likewise, people with impaired vision should request the help of others to regularly examine their feet to ensure good foot health.

In the event of an ulcer developing, treatment interventions need to be initiated promptly and appropriately, with the aim to close the foot ulcer as quickly as possible. This is needed to help prevent potential recurrence, reduce the risk of secondary infection developing and limit the need for lower-extremity amputation (Kravitz et al. 2007).

The effective treatment of neuropathic foot ulcers requires a thorough understanding of the factors linked to the development of chronic wounds of the foot. It is for this reason that all people with diabetes, including those in the very early stages of foot problems, should be referred without delay to a specialist podiatry team for assessment, intervention and education.

Painful neuropathy

Many people who develop neuropathy do not experience pain; however, in those who do, pain is a distressing complication of DSP and can be the main factor that prompts the person with diabetes to seek medical help and advice. Patients describe their pain using various terms including 'burning', 'pins and needles', 'shooting', 'cramping', and also a feeling of hypersensitivity, particularly to the bedclothes at night time. People also complain that they experience the feeling of walking on pebbles, cotton wool or scalding sand.

The severity and distribution of the pain differs between people. Some may have mild symptoms in one or two toes, while others have continuous pain in both legs that radiates to the upper limbs (Tesfaye and Kempler 2005).

The onset of pain can be acute and commonly occurs in those with type 1 diabetes who experience very poor glycaemic control over a period of time. Acute pain can also develop following a rapid improvement in blood glucose control after initiation of intensive treatment. Fortunately, in acute painful neuropathies the symptoms have been known to resolve themselves within a year.

Chronic pain is more commonly reported than acute pain and is associated with DSP. The presence of unpleasant sensory symptoms and pain builds up over a period of weeks and leads to persistent burning pain in the lower limbs and an associated 'dead' feeling. These symptoms are often exacerbated at night making it difficult for the person to gain adequate rest and sleep.

Treatment of neuropathic pain

Treatment of neuropathic pain is complicated and often ineffectual. A thorough medical history and examination needs to be undertaken to exclude other possible causes of leg pain such as prolapsed intervertebral disc, spinal canal stenosis or lumbar–sacral nerve root compression (Tesfaye and Kempler 2005). Once painful DSP has been confirmed, the pharmacological treatment currently available is often complicated with unwanted, unpleasant side-effects that are generally not outweighed by the pharmacological benefits.

Tablet treatments currently available include the use of tricyclic compounds, which are used in low-dose form as first-line agents. These drugs have been used to replace traditional analgesics for many years, but many patients fail to gain any pain or symptomatic relief from them. The anticonvulsants gabapentin and pregabalin are also often used and tend to be better tolerated with fewer side-effects than the tricyclic compounds, but again their value in reducing neuropathic pain is negligible.

Alternative pain relief measures have been researched in attempts to improve the pain-related outcomes of these people. Bosi *et al.* (2005) considered the effectiveness of frequency-modulated electromagnetic neural stimulation (FREMS) in the treatment of painful diabetic neuropathy. Their study reported that pain measured by patients using a visual analogue scale was significantly reduced during the daytime and at night-time when they underwent FREMS. Furthermore, treatment by FREMS significantly increased the person's sensory tactile perception, assessed by the use of a monofilament, thus potentially reducing the incidence of further foot damage due to lack of sensation. Follow-up measurements 4 months after treatment revealed that the initial benefits had been maintained, with an additional reported quality of life improvement.

Transcutaneous electrical nerve stimulation (TENS), which has been used for different types of pain relief for many years, was specifically compared to high-frequency external muscle stimulation (HF) in the treatment of painful DSP (Reichstein *et al.* 2005). In comparing the two treatment modalities in people with type 2 diabetes who had developed DSP, Reichstein *et al.* (2005) report that HF is more effective than TENS in relieving the symptoms of both non-painful and painful neuropathy.

Both studies offer novel, alternative approaches to the treatment of DSP, and while the results are encouraging, they need to be confirmed in larger, multicentre, long-term randomized controlled trials. Nevertheless, they offer new hope to patients with DSP, who are more than aware of the difficulties in treating the condition.

Case study: Malcolm

Malcolm is a 64-year-old man who has had type 2 diabetes for the past 15 years. Six months ago he treated himself to a pair of new walking boots to wear while out walking through fields with his dog. After wearing the new boots for 10 days he was putting on a pair of socks and noticed, by chance, an ulcer on the apex of his big toe, on the plantar surface. It was not painful and did not appear to be infected, so he cleaned it with some antiseptic solution and applied a simple Elastoplast® dressing.

He was not unduly worried about the ulcer and as it was not causing him any pain or discomfort. He tried to keep the wound clean, dry and covered with an adhesive dressing. He also continued to wear his new walking boots, as they appeared comfortable and supportive and he did not associate the boots with the cause of the ulcer.

After 3 weeks of treating the ulcer himself, Malcolm became increasingly concerned as it did not appear to be healing and his foot was becoming red and swollen around the ulcer site. He decided to make an appointment with his general practitioner (GP) for the following day. The GP ascertains the following information from Malcolm.

Past medical history

- Generally fit and well but has been having more falls recently for no apparent reason.
- Type 2 diabetes for the past 15 years. His last annual review was 2 years ago as he was on a long holiday at the time of his last review and as he felt fine, he did not make an appointment on his return.
- He had laser treatment for diabetic background retinopathy 6 years ago and has had annual retinal photography since. No further complications have been noted.
- He has a blood glucose meter at home but confesses to only measuring his blood glucose level if he is not feeling very well.

Family history

- Retired school teacher.
- Married to Daisy, who is generally fit and well.
- Drinks 4–5 glasses of white wine per week.
- Used to smoke 20 cigarettes per day but gave up completely 18 months ago.
- Height 1.80 m.
- Weight 111 kg.
- Classed as obese, with a body mass index (BMI) of 33.4 kg/m^2.
- Waist measurement 109 cm.
- Mother died aged 87 years with carcinoma of the stomach.
- Father died age 77 years with congestive heart failure and had poorly controlled type 2 diabetes.

Medication

- Metformin 1 g with breakfast and 1 g with evening meal.
- Pioglitazone 30 mg daily.
- Glipizide 10 mg daily.
- Simvastatin 40 mg at night.

Allergies

- None known.

Examination

- Toes on both feet are clawed, but this is more marked on the left foot.
- Ulcer on apex of big toe on plantar pressure site on left foot, 1 cm in diameter, red and swollen, with no evidence of tissue granulation around the edges.
- Wound oozing yellow pus.
- Callus on plantar pressure surface of second toe on left foot.
- Both feet feel warm, well perfused and with bounding pulses.
- Sweating is diminished and the skin on both feet is dry and flaky.
- The arch of both feet is abnormally raised.
- Diminished sensation in both feet when measured with a 10 g monofilament.
- Blood pressure   140/85 mmHg.
- Pulse   136 bpm, regular.
- Temperature   38.1°C.
- Respirations   15/minute.
- Random capillary blood glucose level   18.4 mmol/l.
- HbA1c   10.4%.

Discussion of Malcolm's case

Based upon the information retrieved, the GP has no hesitation in admitting Malcolm to a medical ward at the local hospital for specialist treatment. The development of a foot ulcer in people with diabetes is classed as a pivotal event that requires urgent and aggressive treatment. The aim is to heal all ulcers within the first 6 weeks of their development.

The key point to consider in this case study is that Malcolm has a long history of type 2 diabetes which, despite a cocktail of different antidiabetes medications, remains poorly controlled. This is evidenced by the high random capillary blood glucose level of 18.4 mmol/l (normal range 4–7 mmol/l) taken in the GP's surgery, and the high HbA1c level (normal range 6.5–7.5%). This indicates that Malcolm's glycaemic control has been poor for quite some time and as a devastating consequence he has developed peripheral neuropathy. There are also clear links between the neuropathy and the retinopathy with which Malcolm was diagnosed 6 years ago. Both conditions develop from microvascular changes that occur as a result of prolonged hyperglycaemia. As Malcolm has not attended an annual review for 2 years he could have had the neuropathy for some time and has not taken active steps to bring his blood glucose levels under control, which would have helped to halt or reduce the neuropathy's rate of progression.

Malcolm has commented to the GP that he has been falling more frequently for no apparent reason. Fortunately, to date he has not seriously injured himself as a result of a fall. Falls in patients with diabetes may be an indication of peripheral, as well as central, neurological dysfunction in that they do not have full spatial awareness of where their lower limbs are. This gives them an altered and disordered gait that impedes mobility and makes falls more likely. The presence of diabetes alone increases a person's risk of hospitalization due to a fall by 1.8 times compared to those who do not have diabetes (Bloomgarden 2007).

This information is therefore important, as it helps to confirm the diagnosis of neuropathy. The potential discomfort and consequences of frequent falls may be the impetus the person needs to ensure blood glucose levels are maintained between 4 and 7 mmol/l over prolonged periods to help prevent the neuropathy developing further.

Up to 35% of all patients with diabetes will have asymptomatic neuropathy (Edmonds and Foster 2000), which will only be detected by clinical examination. An important clinical sign in diagnosing neuropathy is that the patient does not complain of any pain, even when significant foot ulcers are present. The apex of the toe on the plantar surface is the prime area in which neuropathic foot ulcers develop. In these people, changes in foot structure occur and a claw toe deformity develops leading to the formation of a callus on the plantar pressure site. The increased pressure that results from the callus, if left untreated, eventually causes the skin in the surrounding area to break down (Edmonds and Foster 2000).

On admission to the ward and having been seen by a specialist podiatry team, the diagnosis of neuropathy is confirmed for Malcolm. The ulcer which has now become infected has been exacerbated by poorly fitting walking shoes. This represents a typical case of a person with neuropathy who buys new shoes and is unable to feel where they may be rubbing and causing foot damage. This scenario provides another reason why it is crucial that people with diabetes are positively encouraged to inspect their feet each day, particularly when new footwear has been purchased and used.

Stages of the diabetic foot

Edmonds and Foster (2000) describe a classification system used to stage the diabetic foot. Malcolm's neuropathic foot ulcer would be classed as a stage 3 becoming grade 4. The stages as described by Edmonds and Foster (2000) are shown in Table 4.1.

Treating the neuropathic foot ulcer

Kravitz et al. (2007) highlight some key therapeutic objectives in managing any plantar ulcer. These include the need to:

- maintain a moist wound environment,
- redistribute load in the areas of greatest pressure,
- prevent infection,
- achieve and maintain metabolic control,
- ensure adequate nutritional status,
- initiate appropriate wound care, which will include the removal of necrotic or non-viable tissue,
- promote patient education and compliance.

Table 4.1   Stages of the diabetic foot (Edmonds and Foster 2000).

Stage	General condition
1	The foot is not at risk. The patient does not have any of the risk factors associated with neuropathy, ischaemia, deformity, callus or swelling.
2	The patient has developed at least one of the risk factors for ulceration. This can be divided into the neuropathic or neuroischaemic foot.
3	There is an area on the foot in which the skin has broken down. This usually presents as an ulcer, but blisters, grazes or splits in the skin have a tendency to develop into ulcers. Ulceration is on the plantar surface in the neuropathic foot and on the margin in the neuroischaemic foot.
4	The ulcer has become infected and cellulitis is usually present.
5	Necrosis has developed. In the neuroischaemic foot this is usually secondary to infection; however, ischaemia can also cause necrosis.
6	The foot has become so damaged that it cannot be saved and major amputation is required.

Once the ulcer has healed, management should focus on the prevention of further ulcers developing.

Edmonds and Foster (2000) also identify six main components, which all need to be addressed if Malcolm's foot ulcer is to have any chance of healing. They are:

- mechanical control,
- wound control,
- microbiological control,
- vascular control,
- metabolic control,
- educational control.

Furthermore, a dedicated multidisciplinary approach is crucial and should involve podiatrists, diabetologists, dietitians and nurses. It is vital that all of the multidisciplinary team have a clear understanding of the goals to be achieved and the time frame in which they are to be met. It is also essential that all the members of the team work together to provide a cohesive approach to Malcolm's care. Malcolm also has an important role to play in ensuring that his blood glucose levels are maintained within normal limits for significant periods of time in order to improve his long-term HbA1c reading and thus reduce the development of further complications.

1. Mechanical control

The specialist podiatry team will take responsibility for improving the mechanical control of the foot. Ideally, ulcers must be managed with rest, and pressure should be avoided at all costs; however, to be totally non-weight bearing for a period of time is often difficult for the person to achieve. A range of ambulatory methods have been designed and developed to redistribute plantar pressure in the neuropathic foot. These include specialist footwear, casts, foam wedges, heel protector splints and insoles. More general measures, such as the use of crutches, wheelchairs and zimmer frames, should also be encouraged. The podiatrist will determine which approach is most suitable for Malcolm but, wherever possible, the application of a cast is the most efficient way to relieve plantar pressure. Various casts are currently available and include Aircast®, Total-contact® cast and Scotchcast® boot.

The Aircast® and Scotchcast® boot are removable so that patients can check their ulcers and remove the cast when they go to bed. The Total-contact® cast is permanent and should only be used when the ulcer has failed to respond to the other two types of cast. However, there are potential dangers to using the Total-contact® cast on a foot that is insensitive and painless as there is always the fear of causing further damage to the foot by the cast. With all casts, the patient is at a greatly increased risk of developing further problems due to rubbing, pressure sores and trauma caused by the cast, which can go undetected. All patients are therefore advised to monitor their body temperature and blood glucose levels at least daily to observe for any signs of developing infection, which may have detrimental consequences.

The casts can often be heavy and uncomfortable, reducing a person's mobility and resulting in a high incidence of non-compliance with the treatment. In addition, people may develop 'cast phobia' in which they refuse to wear them. Wearing a cast creates a disparity in the length of the person's legs, which can cause problems in their knee, hip and spine. This can be prevented by raising the shoe on the opposite side. There is also danger of sustaining a fracture or Charcot foot developing if the person walks too far and too soon after having the cast removed (Edmonds and Foster 2000). Patient education is therefore vital in this incidence.

2. Wound control

Wound control should also be under the auspices of the podiatry team and will be based around the regular debridement of the wound, generally with forceps and a scalpel. This is the preferred method of surgical removal of non-viable tissue (Kravitz et al. 2007).

Debridement of the wound will include removing the callus, which in turn will lower plantar pressures and enable a complete assessment of the ulcer and its margins. Healing is also encouraged with debridement, as a chronic wound is surgically turned into an acute wound and the healing process is retriggered. This also facilitates the drainage of exudates and removal of dead tissue, which helps to prevent infection from occurring. It also assists in the effective treatment of an underlying infection, as in Malcolm's situation.

Other techniques to facilitate debridement and promote healing include the use of lavatherapy, skin grafts and a vacuum-assisted closure pump, which applies gentle negative pressure to the ulcer. This enriches the blood supply to the area and stimulates granulation of the wound.

Sterile non-adhesive dressings should be used to cover all open diabetic foot lesions to help protect the foot from further trauma, absorb exudate and reduce the risk of infection and thus promote healing. Dressings should be carefully lifted every day to observe the wound and facilitate early detection of any further complications (Edmonds and Foster 2000).

3. Microbiological control

Foot ulcers are open wounds that provide a perfect portal for pathogens to enter, leading to the development of infection. If infection is left untreated, it can threaten the viability of the limb and ultimately the person's life.

Infection should be suspected if there is purulent drainage from the wound, significant necrotic tissue and the possible presence of a sinus track, which is associated with a deeper abscess. The ability to probe bone within the open wound, or bone that is visible at the wound site, provides the practitioner with a clear indication that the wound has become infected. In addition, ascending cellulitis, which is present in Malcolm's case, is depicted by the redness and swelling of the foot and limb, and a general feeling of malaise. An abnormally high temperature can be a sign that immediate hospitalization and aggressive treatment is required (Kravitz et al. 2007).

While the value of antibiotics used prophylactically in the non-infected foot has not been established, they should certainly be prescribed in the presence of infection. In Malcolm's case, wound swabs will need to be taken and he should be prescribed a broad-spectrum antibiotic without hesitation. As most diabetic foot ulcers are polymicrobial, a diet of different antibiotics may be required based upon the results from the wound swabs; a combination of oral and intravenous antibiotics may be needed. Wound swabs should be repeated after 4–6 weeks and the prescribed antibiotic prescription amended to take account of the new wound swab cultures (Kravitz *et al.* 2007).

4. Vascular control

All persons with foot problems related to diabetes, including Malcolm, will need to be assessed for the presence of ischaemia to determine whether there is an adequate vascular supply to the wound to promote healing. One way to detect the presence of ischaemia is via assessment using the Doppler waveform, if available. As mentioned previously, the use of the ankle–brachial index, which can indicate the presence of claudication and critical limb ischaemia, is not a reliable marker in people with diabetes.

Transcutaneous oxygen tension is a non-invasive method for monitoring arterial oxygen tension and reflects the level of arterial perfusion in the limb. A level below 30 mmHg indicates severe ischaemia but it must be recognized that levels can be falsely lowered in the presence of oedema and cellulitis (Edmonds and Foster 2000).

In recognizing the serious nature of foot ulceration, Khaodhiar *et al.* (2007) tested the efficacy of medical hyperspectral technology (HT) in predicting foot ulcer healing. While the ankle–brachial index and transcutaneous oxygen tension can determine the level of ischaemia, they are not able to predict wound healing. Previously, the only way to do this was to measure changes to the ulcer over a 4-week period of intensive treatment. This technique yields mixed results in terms of efficacy and requires sequential patient examinations, which are inconvenient, costly and may delay the initiation of appropriate therapy.

Medical hyperspectral technology measures the levels of oxyhaemoglobin and deoxyhaemoglobin at, or near to the ulcer area and on the upper and lower extremity distant from the ulcer. Based on these readings an HT healing index for each site is calculated. Positive conclusions have been drawn from the research by Khaodhiar *et al.* (2007) on the ability of HT to identify microvascular abnormalities and predict ulcer healing as well as measuring tissue oxygenation, which is so vital in the healing process. A limitation of the study is the small sample size used to gain the data (37 patients with 21 ulcer sites); however, as the researchers acknowledge, statistically relevant results were obtained regardless, indicating the power and usefulness of this medical interaction.

If, after 6 weeks of intensive optimal treatment, the healing of the ulcer has not progressed in a positive direction then angiography should seriously be considered. This is a worthwhile treatment to improve arterial blood flow and aid healing, but if the lesions are too widespread for angiography to be effective, then angioplasty could be a viable option. This is a major operation, not without its risks, and therefore should not be entered into lightly (Edmonds and Foster 2000).

5. Metabolic control

Excellent glycaemic control and adequate nutritional intake is needed if the ulcer has any chance of healing. In order to assess this, Malcolm will require a full blood count to exclude the presence of anaemia and will also require measurement of his serum electrolytes and serum creatinine to assess his renal function. Serum albumin levels should also be obtained as an indicator of Malcolm's nutrition level. A recording of <3.5 g/dl would indicate malnutrition, which would need to be corrected.

Hyperglycaemia can impair wound healing and neutrophil function, therefore it is vital to maintain Malcolm's blood glucose level between the normal parameters of 4–7 mmol/l at all times. As previously mentioned, Malcolm's random blood glucose reading and high HbA1c, in addition to the development of background retinopathy and now a neuropathic foot ulcer, indicate that his blood glucose level has probably been poor and out of the acceptable range for some time. Reassessment of glycaemic control is therefore needed and should focus on dietary aspects, current pharmacological management and lifestyle issues.

Dietary aspects

As part of the multidisciplinary approach to Malcolm's care, he would need to be referred to a dietitian for specific advice on maintaining good nutrition levels in order to enhance the healing process. It will also be important for healthcare professionals to ensure that Malcolm receives a healthy and nutritionally balanced diet during his stay in hospital.

Malcolm will also require information on how to make 'healthy' food choices that will minimize the impact on his blood glucose levels. It would be appropriate for him to be advised upon and encouraged to follow a low glycaemic index (GI) diet, which will help to prevent large glucose excursions throughout the day. As this diet plan draws on the principles of healthy eating and maintaining the feeling of satiety for longer, this may also have positive benefits in helping Malcolm to lose weight as he will feel less hungry and the urge to 'snack' will be lessened, thus reducing his overall calorie intake. However, the need for a nutritionally balanced diet to aid healing cannot be emphasized strongly enough and should be a priority. Any associated weight loss would be seen as a bonus but should not take priority.

Current pharmacological management

The current antidiabetes medication that Malcolm is taking needs to be reviewed, as it clearly is not able to maintain adequate blood glucose levels. Ordinarily it may be possible for someone who has poor diabetes control to amend their diet and lifestyle and as a result gain glycaemic control, but in Malcolm's case as he has a neuropathic foot ulcer that needs to be treated promptly and effectively, there is no time to wait to monitor the effects of diet and lifestyle changes on blood glucose control. Diet and lifestyle changes would still be positively encouraged, but would need to be coupled with changes in his medication regimen.

Malcolm is currently taking a range of antidiabetes medication including metformin, pioglitazone and glipizide, all of which work in slightly different ways to reduce blood glucose levels (see Chapter 2). In view of this, there are two main options open to Malcolm with regards to his pharmacological management.

Option 1 is to review and maintain oral antidiabetes medication. The underlying principle in this option is to recognize that the current tablets and doses are not sufficient to maintain blood glucose levels within healthy limits. Malcolm is not currently taking the maximum recommended dose of metformin, therefore one option would be to increase the metformin from 2 g to the maximum permitted dose of 3 g per day if he is able to tolerate it gastrointestinally. Malcolm needs to take this in two to three divided doses with his main meals of the day but the effects of this dose increase may not be reflected in his blood glucose levels for 4–8 weeks. In addition, the pioglitazone could also be increased from 30 mg to 45 mg daily, if tolerated, but again the effects on his blood glucose level may not be seen immediately due to the longevity of the drug action.

Finally, an increase in glipizide doses could also be initiated to a maximum dose of 20 mg daily divided into two doses to be taken before breakfast and the other main meal of the day. While there are other potential drug options that could be commenced, experience has not shown these to be particularly effective at the late stage in the disease process that Malcolm is at.

Option 2 is to commence insulin therapy. While it is certainly possible to prescribe maximum doses of the three main antidiabetes medications for Malcolm, as mentioned, the effects of these may not be seen for a few weeks. Time is of the essence in trying to heal an ulcer and therefore a preferred option in this case would be to commence Malcolm on insulin therapy.

Key point

Insulin therapy should result in the:

- Abolition of symptoms.
- Maintenance of ideal body weight without causing excessive weight gain.
- Optimization of glucose control – without making the person obsessional.
- Prevent complications or delay the progress existing problems.

As control is needed quickly, the use of a once-a-day long-acting insulin such as Levemir® or Lantus® would not be a preferred option as results from this regimen are variable. A twice-a-day mixed insulin taken before breakfast and evening meal or a four-times-a-day basal/bolus regimen would be advised, depending on Malcolm's preference and his current lifestyle.

When commencing insulin therapy, the current pioglitazone and glipizide would be discontinued, particularly as pioglitazone is contraindicated with the use of insulin. As Malcolm is overweight and likely to be insulin resistant, a decision to maintain the metformin may be taken. This works on the principle that it will enhance the action of the injected insulin, resulting in potentially smaller doses of insulin being needed thus reducing the risk of unwanted weight gain.

The initial insulin dose is calculated by giving 0.5–1 unit of insulin per kilogram of body weight. Therefore, as Malcolm is 111 kg he will need between 55 and 111 units of insulin per day. The higher amount would be opted for, as he is overweight and potentially insulin resistant but the dose can be titrated up according to Malcolm's needs.

If commencing a twice-daily insulin regimen, the 111 units of insulin would be divided up into two doses equalling two-thirds of the units given before breakfast and the remaining third given before his evening meal. An example prescription could therefore be:

NovoMix®30 insulin, 74 units before breakfast and 37 units before his evening meal.

Alternatively, on a four-injections-a-day basal/bolus insulin regimen, the 111 units would be divided 50% basal insulin and 50% bolus insulin, divided into the number of meals eaten and the amount of carbohydrate at each meal time. A typical prescription depicting this insulin regimen would be:

Glargine insulin, 55 units to be taken in one injection at the same time each day.

NovoRapid® or Humalog® insulin: 15 units with breakfast, 18 units with lunch and 23 units with main evening meal.

These doses would be titrated to take into account the amount and type of carbohydrate Malcolm is eating at each mealtime and his levels of insulin resistance, as well as the amount of exercise/activity he is undertaking.

Key point

In the above example, the healthcare professional would need to ensure that the insulin pens prescribed to administer the above doses can deliver the insulin in 1-unit increments rather then the usual 2-unit increments.

For both of the above potential insulin regimens, the figures given are based upon 'rule of thumb' and educated trial and error. They provide a starting point for insulin therapy and will almost certainly have to be amended once the individual reaction is known in order to gain appropriate blood glucose control.

Blood glucose monitoring
In order to assess the efficacy of either of the above options it will be necessary to monitor Malcolm's blood glucose levels on a regular basis. This should be done preprandially, before he has had anything to eat, first thing in a morning. It should then be repeated 2 hours after each of his main meals. This takes into account the expected rise in blood glucose levels with ingestion of food and provides the optimum times to monitor blood glucose levels and consequently ascertain the efficacy of the prescribed treatment.

> **Key point**
>
> If long-term complications of diabetes are to be prevented, blood glucose levels need to be returned to within normal limits 120 minutes after each meal.

Testing blood glucose levels outside of these times does not enable a clear and accurate picture of blood glucose control to be formulated. Once blood glucose control is achieved, then the frequency of blood glucose monitoring can be reduced.

> **Key point**
>
> Amending prescribed treatment regimens should only be done following the identification of 'patterns and trends' in the blood glucose readings taken over a few days and not based upon a single blood glucose reading.

Lifestyle issues
Further weight gain is a potential major factor when considering Malcolm's lifestyle. Despite being overweight, he is obviously quite active walking his dog. As he is now expected to be non-weight bearing on his foot, he is no longer able to exercise and his weight could escalate as a result, increasing his insulin resistance at the same time. This problem could also be exacerbated with the introduction of insulin which, being a growth hormone, has the side-effect of weight gain. Dietary help and support are therefore crucial for Malcolm.

6. Educational control
Educating the person about the causes of foot ulceration, the requirements to promote healing and prevention of further ulceration is of great importance if a positive clinical outcome is to be achieved.

Malcolm needs to be advised in clear terms that foot ulcers have the potential to become a very serious problem for people with diabetes and the fact that many of them are painless makes them more difficult to detect and easier to ignore.

Unfortunately, by the time the patient begins to experience pain due to the ulcer, damage to the foot has reached a critical stage.

Compliance with treatment needs to be emphasized and the more rest the foot can be given, the more effective the healing process will be. Indeed with foot ulcers, every time the patient takes a step it is the equivalent of hitting the ulcer with a hammer (Edmonds and Foster 2000). Malcolm therefore needs to be aware of the value of the special shoes, insoles and plaster casts that he may have been prescribed, as these are designed to take the load off the foot if walking is unavoidable.

The healing process and the need to surgically remove all debris and hard skin needs to be explained and emphasized that this should always be done by a doctor or podiatrist to prevent further damage to the foot. The foot should be carefully inspected daily by the person for signs of any changes such as swelling, increased or altered discharge, a change in colour or an altered pain threshold. Daily inspection of the foot should be continued once the ulcer has healed and the development of any further calluses or lesions should be reported immediately to the GP or specialist podiatry team.

If Malcolm commences on insulin therapy, he will need information regarding the following:

- The type and action of insulin being used.
- Injections sites and the need to rotate these to prevent lipohypertrophy.
- Injection technique.
- Storage of insulin.
- The change in the absorption rate of insulin when injected at different sites and when skin temperature differs.
- The need to inform the UK Driver Vehicle Licensing Agency (DVLA) that he has commenced insulin therapy.
- The risks and treatment of hypoglycaemia.
- Sick day rules.
- The need for careful and appropriate blood glucose monitoring.

If all of the above factors are taken into the consideration and acted upon by both the multidisciplinary healthcare team and the patient, the chances of the ulcer healing within a short space of time will be increased, thus reducing morbidity and mortality rates. Emphasis will then need to be placed on the need to prevent further recurrences; this can be achieved via optimal blood glucose control, diet and lifestyle changes and careful observations of both feet on a daily basis.

Conclusion

In this chapter, the devastating effects of developing neuropathy as a complication of diabetes have been highlighted and emphasized. The different types of peripheral and autonomic neuropathies that can develop in a person with diabetes have been explained, along with how these present themselves. The recognized signs and symptoms of neuropathy have been included to facilitate thorough assessment by the healthcare professional.

In considering the development of neuropathy, the results of the Diabetes Control and Complications Trial (1997) have been drawn upon to highlight the importance of achieving and maintaining good blood glucose control.

Finally, a common complication of diabetic neuropathy is the development of a neuropathic foot ulcer. The prevention, care and management of this has been explored via a case study depicting a typical scenario seen in many podiatry out-patient clinics and hospital wards.

5

Diabetes and the surgical patient

Aims of the chapter

This chapter will:

1. Critically consider the effects of anaesthesia and surgery on metabolic and blood glucose control.
2. Discuss the implications for practice when a person with diabetes is kept nil by mouth and is stressed due to the anaesthetic and surgery, at risk of infection and has reduced eating and drinking and limited mobility.
3. Describe the optimal care and management of a person with diabetes undergoing major abdominal surgery.
4. Consider the implications of emergency and day surgery for people with type 1 and type 2 diabetes in relation to the different antidiabetes treatments currently available.

This chapter details a patient with type 1 diabetes who is admitted to hospital for major abdominal surgery. Patients with diabetes undergo the same type of surgical procedures as people who do not have diabetes, but it is paramount that the healthcare professional looking after the patient with diabetes fully understands the condition and the effects of surgery on the diabetes and blood glucose control. Owing to the nature of diabetes and the long-term complications, people with both type 1 and type 2 diabetes are at an increased likelihood of requiring cardiac procedures, angioplasty, open heart surgery, amputations and eye surgery – all carrying significant risks to the patient.

While major abdominal surgery is not a common complication of diabetes, it has been chosen for the case study as it encompasses a number of significant pre- and postoperative implications for the person with diabetes, such as prolonged episodes of being nil by mouth, nausea and vomiting, surgical incision and postoperative pain. Postoperatively, it does not initially generally require care in an intensive care unit, thus placing the immediate postoperative management in the hands of the surgical ward healthcare team. The principles and practice identified in relation to the patient in the case study in this chapter can also be applied in part, or in full, to other patients with diabetes who require different types of surgical procedures.

Within this chapter, the specific diabetes-related factors that need to be considered during the pre-, intra- and postoperative phases are identified; however, general and routine pre- and postoperative care and management will only be discussed if they cause specific concerns for the patient with diabetes.

Risk of surgery

In times gone by it was widely considered that patients with type 1 or type 2 diabetes were at a significantly increased risk of morbidity and mortality when undergoing major surgery, compared to those who had undergone the same surgical procedure but did not have diabetes. Fortunately, over recent years it has been shown that with good pre-, intra- and postoperative management of the diabetes, these patients are no longer at an increased risk.

Hormonal response

Surgery is a form of major trauma to the body and promotes a neuroendocrine stress response that increases blood glucose levels to provide the person with 'metabolic energy' to overcome the anaesthetic and surgical disturbance to the body. This is achieved by stimulating an increase in the secretion of stress hormones such as adrenaline, glucagon, cortisol and growth hormone, all of which act to raise blood glucose levels by effecting glucogenolysis and gluconeogenesis in the liver. The damaging effects of peripheral insulin resistance, impaired insulin secretion and increased fat and protein breakdown are unfortunately also features of the increased levels of stress hormones (Marks 2003). The magnitude of this neuroendocrine response is determined by the severity of the surgery and the presence of complications such as infection, bleeding, acidosis and hypotension.

People who do not have diabetes are able to react to the rising blood glucose levels by automatically secreting more insulin, but for the person with diabetes this is not possible and during surgery and hospitalization the fine balance of blood glucose control has to be maintained by a healthcare professional. The responsibility of this is great, particularly while the person is under anaesthesia. A person with type 1 diabetes is at risk of developing diabetic ketoacidosis (DKA) and a person with type 2 diabetes has an increased susceptibility to the detrimental effects of hyperglycaemia and potentially to hyperosmolar, non-ketotic acidosis (HONK).

It is for these reasons that, wherever possible, surgical procedures on patients with diabetes are performed under local or spinal anaesthesia. Although a rise in stress hormone secretion will still be evident with these types of anaesthesia, it tends to generate less of an effect on catabolism. This lesser response enables greater metabolic control to be achieved, thus reducing the risks for the patient. Local and spinal anaesthesia is also associated with a lower incidence of nausea and vomiting, which makes maintaining blood glucose control within the target of 4–7 mmol/l more achievable. In addition, if the person is awake during the procedure they are able to identify the signs of an impending hypoglycaemic episode and seek appropriate help.

Case study: Julie

Julie is a 51-year-old woman who developed Crohn's disease in her colon approximately 10 years ago. Since her diagnosis, the condition has become increasingly more difficult to control and the time she spends in remission is reducing.

During relapse periods, Julie complains of quite severe pain in the lower right side of her abdomen with associated diarrhoea mixed with mucus and, at times, blood. She also often experiences tenesmus – the feeling of wanting to go to the toilet but with nothing to pass. During each relapse she generally feels unwell with a loss of appetite resulting in weight loss, fever and tiredness. These symptoms are complicated further by the presence of type 1 diabetes making blood glucose control difficult, putting Julie at increased risk of developing hypo- or hyperglycaemia.

Over the years, different and increasing medications have been used on Julie including Salazopyrin® and steroid therapy, but it has reached the point where she is no longer responding effectively to the medication. In the past year, she has had three episodes of hospitalization requiring intravenous steroid therapy, fluid balance and parenteral nutrition. It has now been concluded that surgery to remove the area of diseased bowel is the only option for Julie, particularly as the condition is also impacting negatively on her diabetes control.

Julie has been admitted to the surgical ward for an elective resection and anastomosis surgical procedure. She is currently quite well and is not enduring an acute bout of Crohn's disease.

Past medical history

- Type 1 diabetes diagnosed when she was 13 years of age.
- Crohn's disease 10 years ago, aged 41 years.
- Laparoscopic cholecystectomy 2 years ago for gallstones thought to be secondary to the Crohn's disease.
- Smoked approximately 15–20 cigarettes per day from the age of 20 years until she gave up 5 years ago when she became aware of the detrimental link between smoking and Crohn's disease.

Continued

Family history

- Both parents are still alive and in their late 70s.
- Her father has generally been fit and well up until about 2 years ago, when he developed angina. This is largely under control with pharmacological medication.
- Julie's mother was diagnosed with Crohn's disease when she was 39 years old. She is fortunate in that she has quite long periods of remission and usually responds well to steroid therapy during episodes of acute inflammation.
- Julie has one younger sister who has also recently developed Crohn's disease.

Medication

- Salazopyrin® 1 g four times a day.
- Prednisolone 20 mg twice daily during an acute relapse of her Crohn's.
- Lantus® insulin, 32 units taken at 10 p.m.
- NovoRapid® insulin, 8 units with breakfast, 10 units with lunch and 15 units with evening meal.

Allergies

- None known.

Examination

- Blood pressure   130/70 mmHg.
- Pulse   88 bpm, regular.
- Temperature   37.4°C.
- Respirations   14/minute.
- Random capillary blood glucose level   8.2 mmol/l.
- HbA1c   6.4%.
- Weight   65 kg.
- Body mass index (BMI)   25.7 kg/m².

Discussion of Julie's case

Diabetes care, management and control is always made more difficult where there are co-existing conditions that affect the absorption of carbohydrates and the speed at which the food is transported through the gastrointestinal system; one such condition is Crohn's disease. The erratic absorption of food will undoubtedly impact on glycaemic control, making it difficult for the person to predict when blood glucose levels will rise and what their actual insulin requirements will be. In addition, during an acute exacerbation of Crohn's disease the person does not feel well enough to eat, which again makes diabetes control and managing insulin requirements very difficult.

In Julie's case, her diabetes control can be assessed via the random blood glucose capillary measurement taken on admission to the ward. This indicates that at the moment in time when the blood sample was taken the measurement was just above the required level of 4–7 mmol/l. From this, it can be safely assumed that Julie is not hypoglycaemic and the risk of her being ketotic is low. Little else can be gained from this result. It is an isolated example and a more in-depth blood glucose profile would be needed to identify patterns and trends in blood glucose control, which may be rather complicated due to the poor absorption of food.

The haemoglobin A1c (HbA1c) result has more significance in considering long-term blood glucose control. Julie's result is currently just under the normal parameters of 6.5–7.5%. While this is encouraging and on the surface indicates that Julie has excellent diabetes control, it must also be considered in relation to her Crohn's disease. A low HbA1c can also be an indicator of recurrent hypoglycaemic events, which could be linked to the erratic absorption of carbohydrates that Julie will experience as a result of Crohn's disease.

In people with diabetes who do not have disorders of the gastrointestinal tract, it is expected that, on average, the carbohydrate intake of a meal will be largely absorbed within 2 hours of eating the food. During these 2 hours, blood glucose levels will rise and should then return back to within normal limits at the end of this time period. The usual controlled absorption of carbohydrate in the gastro-intestinal tract makes predicting when blood glucose levels will rise and fall relatively straightforward, thus enabling the person with diabetes to calculate their insulin requirements. Indeed, a number of insulin preparations currently available, e.g. NovoRapid®, Humalog®, NovoMix® 30 and Humalog® 25, all have an action time that mimics the expected 2-hour rise and fall in blood glucose levels.

When gastrointestinal tract disorders are put into the equation with diabetes, the absorption of the carbohydrate and blood glucose rise cannot be predicted, making it very difficult for the person to be able to match his or her insulin action to rising blood glucose levels. As a result the insulin, once injected, will become effective regardless of the person's blood glucose level; this can lead to severe hypoglycaemia if no, or less than the anticipated, carbohydrate is absorbed at the same time. A regulated absorption of carbohydrate is needed to counteract a fall in blood glucose levels due to the action of the insulin.

Conversely, to avoid hypoglycaemia, the amount of insulin injected may be reduced if carbohydrate absorption is expected to be suboptimal. In this situation, carbohydrate absorption is good but there are insufficient circulating levels of insulin, rendering the person at risk of hyperglycaemia and diabetic ketoacidosis.

Similar difficulties matching insulin requirements with rising blood glucose levels will also be encountered by the person who is prescribed sulphonylureas for diabetes control. The extra insulin produced as a result of the sulphonylurea may not occur at the time the carbohydrate is absorbed, resulting in potentially detrimental high or low blood glucose levels.

A further impediment in Julie's case that makes her increasingly less able to control her diabetes is that she has a low-grade pyrexia, suggesting an inflammatory process is occurring within the bowel. The presence of inflammation causes the autonomic nervous system to exhibit a stress response, which results in the release of adrenaline, cortisol, growth hormone and adrenocorticotrophic hormone (ACTH). As mentioned previously, all of these act to increase blood glucose levels as in the fight or flight scenario, and the difficulties of maintaining glycaemic control throughout this process are compounded.

Preoperative assessment

All patients with diabetes undergoing elective surgery require a detailed and comprehensive preoperative assessment. In addition to the general assessment for anyone undergoing surgery, the person with diabetes needs to be carefully assessed for specific complications of diabetes that may impact on the care and management required during this time. These include the presence of: (1) peripheral and autonomic neuropathy; (2) obesity and the metabolic syndrome; and (3) metabolic control.

1. Peripheral and autonomic neuropathy

As stated in Chapter 4, neuropathy is a common complication in patients with type 1 and type 2 diabetes and can affect a number of different body systems. For the patient undergoing surgery, the presence of peripheral neuropathy should be ascertained as extra vigilance needs to be given in preventing the development of pressure sores. Neuropathy can cause the patient to have diminished sensory feeling and he or she may be unable to feel pressure that would usually trigger a change in position. The patient therefore needs to be educated on the importance of regular movement and position changes, particularly in the postoperative period when mobility will be more limited.

Gastroparesis is an autonomic neuropathic disorder induced by diabetes that needs to be identified in the preoperative phase. A definitive diagnosis of gastroparesis can be difficult to obtain but the condition should be firmly suspected in persons who are known to have erratic blood glucose readings, particularly postprandially, and have developed other complications of diabetes. Diabetes longevity is a less-reliable predictor of gastroparesis, unlike the development of diabetic retinopathy and diabetic neuropathy.

The reported incidence of gastroparesis ranges from 9.9 to 76% and is thought to increase the person's gastric fluid volume despite preoperative starving. This causes an increased risk of aspiration and vomiting during and after surgery (Jellish *et al.* 2005). For this reason a number of anaesthetists will prescribe metoclopramide prophylactically in patients with diabetes to reduce gastric residual volumes and therefore reduce the risk of gastric aspiration.

In considering this practice and highlighting the potentially adverse effects of metoclopramide, Jellish *et al.* (2005) conducted research on the level of fasting residual gastric volumes in patients with diabetes. They found that even in people with diabetes and multiple co-morbidities, the residual gastric volumes after preoperative fasting were minimal and, while metoclopramide was effective in reducing these volumes further, the changes were inconsequential. In the light of the data collected, Jellish *et al.* (2005) do not advocate the use of prokinetic agents such as metoclopramide to reduce gastric volumes in people with well-controlled diabetes; however, they do state the need for these patients to fast for more than 8 hours preoperatively. This obviously has implications on maintaining appropriate metabolic control in people with diabetes for a longer time preoperatively. Jellish *et al.* (2005) also suggest that metoclopramide may still be indicated in those with poorly controlled diabetes, evidenced by an HbA1c result greater than 9%.

As peripheral neuropathy can mask the normal crushing pain experienced when a person has a myocardial infarction (MI), this can occur but be undiagnosed and the person does not seek help. A patient who has a history of a recent MI within the 3 months prior to surgery has a 6% rate of reinfarction or death if surgery is performed. The rate falls to a 2% chance of reinfarction or death if the surgery is performed within 6 months of the initial MI. Even if surgery can be, and is, delayed until a period of 6 months or more has lapsed since the MI, the person is still at a 1.5% risk of reinfarction or death due to the surgery (Goldman 1995). In response to this, the healthcare team, including the anaesthetist, need to be vigilant in assessing the person for potential cardiac complications such as ischaemia and/or 'silent' MI.

2. Obesity and the metabolic syndrome

Unfortunately, we are in the midst of an obesity epidemic, which is one of the largest health challenges currently facing the UK. According to the statistics produced by Diabetes UK (2005), the obesity rate in adult women and men has nearly trebled in the past 22 years and now affects over one in five adults in the UK. As a consequence, there is a steady and progressive increase in the number of people undergoing bariatric surgery in a drastic attempt to lose weight, but frequently these people have also developed diabetes due to their obesity, which will significantly impact on their clinical outcomes post-surgery.

Obesity on its own has been linked with an increased risk of postoperative wound infection, but when obesity is combined with diabetes there is an elevated risk of the person developing respiratory failure, atrial and ventricular arrhythmias, renal impairment and wound infections in the postoperative period (Neligan and Fleisher 2006).

In terms of increased surgical morbidity and mortality, there appears to be two different groups of obese people (Neligan and Fleisher 2006): the 'metabolically healthy, but obese' group and the 'metabolically obese'. The metabolically healthy group are classified as having a BMI >30 kg/m^2 but do not have such conditions as diabetes, hypertension or hyperlipidaemia. The 'metabolically obese' group are classified if they present with two or more of the following abnormalities:

- Type 2 diabetes or impaired glucose tolerance.
- Hypertension – blood pressure >160/90 mmHg.
- Dyslipidaemia – elevated plasma triglyceride (>1.7 mmol/l) and/or high-density lipoprotein (HDL) cholesterol <1.0 mmol/l (female) or <0.9 mmol/l (male).
- Obesity – BMI = 30 kg/m².
- Waist measurement ≥94 cm in men, ≥89 cm in South Asian men and ≥80 cm in women.
- Microalbuminuria.

Little research has been undertaken on the surgical care of patients with the metabolic syndrome, but what is known is that these patients are at an increased risk of developing atherosclerotic cardiovascular events when compared with the 'metabolically healthy but obese' group. The combination of obesity and diabetes causes an increase in systemic inflammation, endothelial dysfunction and thrombogenecity (all of which are explained in further detail in Chapter 6) but impact negatively on surgical morbidity and mortality rates.

It is therefore clear that to reduce the risk of postoperative morbidity and mortality in the metabolically obese cohort of patients they need to be screened, encouraged and motivated to reduce their BMI preoperatively via a diet and exercise programme. In achieving this, their level of hypertension and hyperlipidaemia will also be reduced, but if these measurements are still outside normal parameters pharmacological assistance may need to be prescribed and results stabilized prior to surgery. Fortunately, Julie is not currently classed as obese and therefore her chances of developing the above complications are reduced.

3. Metabolic control

Good glycaemic control pre-, intra- and postoperatively is associated with an increase in positive clinical outcomes and a reduced length of stay in hospital for the patient (Kersten *et al.* 2005). Ouattara *et al.* (2005) considered clinical outcomes and blood glucose control in patients undergoing cardiac surgery; they found that there was a direct positive relationship between higher than normal blood glucose levels during the interoperative period and the risk of severe postoperative morbidity.

In the majority of patients with diabetes undergoing surgery, their glycaemic control will need to be maintained by members of the healthcare team in the immediate pre- and postoperative phase, as well as during the surgery. A fine balance between insulin and dextrose requirements will need to be achieved, but it is recognized that this can be difficult. There are a number of confounding variables such as stress, increased insulin resistance and decreased insulin secretion that will act to disrupt glycaemic control. As mentioned earlier, these patients are at an increased risk of developing DKA or HONK, wound healing is less effective, they are more prone to infection, and hyperglycaemia is thought to exacerbate ischaemic brain damage in the elderly (Haag 2000).

In elective surgical procedures, potential problems relating to poor metabolic control need to be identified and corrected in the weeks leading up to surgery.

This will require the patient to undertake and record intensive self blood glucose monitoring, preprandially and 2 hours after each main meal (IDF 2007). Based upon these recordings, dietary and lifestyle changes may be required in conjunction with a review and possible change in pharmacological treatments. Any changes made to the current treatment plan then need to be re-evaluated for their effectiveness until such a point that the patient has reached optimal, individual metabolic control. This may take a number of weeks to achieve.

Preoperative management

Any patient with diabetes who is to undergo major surgery will require admission to hospital at least the day before the surgery is planned. This will allow the healthcare team to ensure that appropriate glycaemic control is achieved preoperatively to reduce the risks of intra- and postoperative complications. Owing to the extra vigilance that people with diabetes undergoing surgery require, and the increased potential for complications, patients with diabetes should be placed at the beginning of the operating list. This will shorten their preoperative fast and allow the patient to have their operation, return from surgery and be in a stable condition prior to the reduced nursing and medical cover that occurs during the night shift.

1. Bowel management

For Julie, depending on whether or not she will require mechanical bowel preparation, she will need to be admitted to the ward 1–2 days prior to surgery. In considering bowel preparation, there appears to be differing opinions. McCoubrey (2007) considered that primary colonic anastomosis is unsafe to perform without bowel preparation due to the possibility of faecal leakage from the anastomosis causing peritonitis. However, an extensive review by Guenaga et al. (2007) found that there is currently no convincing research to support the use of mechanical bowel preparation and its current use is largely based upon observations and 'expert' opinion. Following a comprehensive, systematic review of the literature, Guenaga et al. (2007) concluded that there was no compelling evidence to suggest that anastomosis leakage occurred and caused complications when bowel preparation had not been administered; however, there was evidence that bowel preparation may in fact increase the likelihood of leakage.

Mechanical bowel preparation can be unpleasant for patients and is associated with complications such as nausea, vomiting, dehydration, hypokalaemia and other electrolyte imbalances. For the person with diabetes these can become life threatening if diabetic ketoacidosis develops as a consequence. In Julie's situation, if mechanical bowel preparation can be avoided this would be favoured, but the decision will be made based upon her consultant's preference.

2. Reduced dietary intake/nil by mouth

During the bowel preparation and preoperatively, Julie will be required to have a reduced dietary intake, and will be nil by mouth in the hours leading up to surgery and in the immediate postoperative period. As a result of this, her glycaemic control will need to be assessed, monitored and amended.

In order to replace Julie's carbohydrate intake while she is on a restricted diet, she will require an intravenous infusion of 10% dextrose, delivered via a pump with a drip counter, at 100 ml/hour. This will act to replace the recommended body requirement of 10 g of carbohydrate per hour (Jerreat 2003). Alternatively, if Julie requires extra fluid intake she could be prescribed 5% dextrose infusion delivered at 200 ml/hour. Her insulin requirements will also need to be altered accordingly, depending on which percentage of dextrose infusion is used.

To control blood glucose levels, an intravenous insulin infusion will be commenced and be given alongside the dextrose infusion. There are currently two schools of thought on how this is best delivered, but any insulin regimen should be able to: (1) ensure good glycaemic control; (2) prevent the occurrence of metabolic disturbances; (3) be easy to understand and follow; and (4) be adaptable to a variety of different situations (Marks 2003).

The safest way to achieve this is via the Alberti regimen, which was described 30 years ago (Alberti and Thomas 1979). Using a 500 ml bag of 10% dextrose solution, 15 units of soluble insulin such as actrapid or Humulin® S and 10 mmol of potassium chloride is added and infused at 100 ml/hour. The blood glucose levels should then be recorded hourly via capillary finger pricks. The amounts of insulin and potassium are altered up or down, depending on the blood glucose and plasma potassium concentrations.

The sliding-scale regimen is a slightly different system for delivering intravenous insulin and dextrose and tends to be currently the most favoured method. This is achieved by the use of two separate infusions attached to the patient via a three-way connector with a non-return valve; 10% dextrose with 10 or 20 mmol of potassium, depending on the person's potassium levels, is infused via one of the connectors and again given at 100 ml/hour.

Insulin and adrenaline stimulate the uptake of potassium into the cells while hyperosmolarity causes potassium to be transported out of the cells into the extracellular spaces. This results in high levels of extracellular potassium but a low blood potassium reading, which needs to be corrected to avoid cardiac arrhythmias. The ideal range for potassium levels is between 4.0 and 5.0 mmol/l but as a result of the above, normal serum potassium levels may not be a true reflection of the total body potassium level.

The second infusion is prepared by diluting 50 units of soluble insulin into 50 ml of normal saline into a syringe, making 1 unit of insulin equal to 1 ml of saline. This is then connected to a syringe pump driver and connected to the patient again through the three-way connector. The rate at which the insulin is infused will be determined by the patient's hourly capillary blood glucose reading (Najarian et al. 2005) with the aim of keeping the blood glucose level between 4 and 7 mmol/l while avoiding hypoglycaemia.

The initial rate of infusion with the sliding-scale regimen can be calculated to give an approximate dose as follows:

Table 5.1 Typical sliding-scale regimen.

Blood glucose (mmol/l)	Insulin infusion rate (units [ml]/hour)
0–4	0.5
4.1–7.0	1
7.1–11.0	2
11.1–17.0	4 (test for ketones if >15 mmol/l)
17.1–22.0	6
>22.0	8 (review regimen)

$$\frac{\text{Blood glucose (mmol/l)}}{5} = \text{units insulin/hour}$$

Sliding-scale regimens differ slightly according to local protocol but a typical sliding-scale infusion rate is shown in Table 5.1.

The two most important things to consider when administering a sliding-scale insulin regimen are:

1. *Never turn off the insulin* – the person always requires a small amount of basal insulin 24 hours per day, every day, for such things as metabolism and cellular energy. If the sliding-scale insulin is switched off, the person becomes completely insulin depleted (unless they are making small amounts of endogenous insulin themselves) within 10–15 minutes, putting them at a greatly increased risk of hyperglycaemia and diabetic ketoacidosis.
2. *Do not let the blood glucose level fall to <4 mmol/l* – allowing the blood glucose level to fall below 4 mmol/l will increase the chances of the insulin infusion being inappropriately switched off and it also puts the patient in a hypoglycaemic state. Once hypoglycaemia is registered by the body, the compensatory mechanism described in Chapter 3 comes into play. This can be very distressing for the person experiencing the 'healthcare-induced hypoglycaemia' and can make gaining optimum blood glucose control more difficult.

If the blood glucose levels are falling, the amount of dextrose being infused should be increased and it may be necessary to maintain blood glucose levels a little higher during this period, e.g. between 6 and 10 mmol/l, to avoid triggering a hypoglycaemic response. Blood glucose levels >10 mmol/l will cause increased diuresis and glycosuria, possible dehydration, hypokalaemia and hyponatraemia. Higher blood glucose levels also cause the blood to become more viscose, leading to problems with clotting and thrombosis (French 2000).

The reason that the Alberti regimen is deemed to be the safest method of the two regimens is because if the intravenous infusion is stopped inadvertently, or the complete bag of 10% dextrose and insulin is infused in a few minutes, there is no risk to the patient of obtaining the substrate without the insulin, or vice versa. With the increased safety and reliability of syringe pumps and via careful assessment and blood glucose monitoring when using a sliding-scale regimen, it could be argued that patient safety is not necessarily compromised.

The disadvantages of the Alberti regimen is that blood glucose control cannot be achieved as accurately as it can be with the sliding-scale regimen. Also, should the insulin or potassium content need to be amended, this would require throwing away the current infusion bag with its contents and a new bag with different amounts of insulin and potassium would need to be made up. This can be time consuming and very wasteful, particularly when insulin requirements change frequently, thus making it a costly exercise.

However, others are quick to point out that the sliding-scale regimen deals with blood glucose levels that have gone before and are now finished with, and it does not treat blood glucose levels prospectively. It therefore appears that an eclectic system drawing on the merits of both regimens is needed for quality blood glucose control.

In view of the sliding-scale insulin being administered and Julie not eating, her usual doses of NovoRapid® with meals will be omitted until she is eating and drinking normally again. Her long-acting Lantus® insulin can, and should, still be given at the same dose as usual; indeed, Najarian *et al.* (2005) and Marks (2003) advocate the use of this practice. As Lantus® has a flat, peakless action, it does not increase the risk of hypoglycaemia and may mean that less insulin needs to be given intravenously. However, the healthcare team should not forget the stress response of the illness and surgery on the body, which will increase insulin requirements and can cause glycaemic control to easily and quickly deteriorate.

In addition to controlling her blood glucose levels, Julie will need to be prepared for theatre in exactly the same way as someone who does not have diabetes. She will need to be nil by mouth according to the local protocol and all oral medications will be ceased on the day of the operation.

Intraoperative management

Currently, there is no proven evidence to suggest benefits of one anaesthetic technique over another in people with diabetes, in terms of mortality or morbidity rates. For many, including those with diabetes, local anaesthesia in which the person remains awake is thought to be preferable as it does not impact as highly on the release of catabolic hormones, making metabolic control easier to achieve and enabling the person to recognize and report the onset of hypoglycaemia. Once the patient has been anaesthetized, they are unable to communicate the signs and symptoms of impending hypoglycaemia, thus placing responsibility on the healthcare professional to prevent such an occurrence.

If hypoglycaemia occurs and is left undetected and untreated, permanent brain damage can result. Also, the body's compensatory response to a declining blood glucose level, which normally acts to raise blood glucose levels, becomes impaired making glycaemic control even more problematic. For these reasons, patients should never undergo anaesthesia without a blood glucose determination before the anaesthetic is given and blood glucose levels should be obtained frequently, at 15-minute intervals throughout the operative procedure.

Obesity, sepsis, steroid administration, poor preoperative metabolic control and a recent episode of diabetic ketoacidosis will act to increase intraoperative insulin requirements (Marks 2003); these factors need to be assessed pre- and intraoperatively so that hyperglycaemia can be avoided during this time.

Hyperglycaemia has been associated with numerous deleterious effects on the myocardium and has been shown to provoke coronary endothelial dysfunction, thus increasing the risk of potentially fatal myocardial ischaemic events (Gross et al. 2003).

Furthermore, patients who return to the ward or intensive care unit from theatre with a history of poor intraoperative glycaemic control prove more difficult for the healthcare team to be able to achieve normalization of glycaemia in the early postoperative period. This often leads to patients experiencing a significantly higher incidence of severe intrahospital morbidity, such as acute renal failure requiring dialysis, septic shock or neurological injury leaving a permanent functional deficit (Ouattara et al. 2005).

Postoperatively, glycaemic control is best achieved via continuation of the sliding-scale insulin regimen that was commenced in the preoperative phase. This will require at least hourly blood glucose recordings with the insulin infusion rate being titrated accordingly.

Autonomic neuropathy predisposes the person with diabetes to intraoperative hypotension, which requires careful and vigilant monitoring as well as the control and treatment of blood pressure and blood volume status (Plodkowski and Edelman 2001). Adequate blood pressure control is also required during this period to ensure renal function is maintained. This can be compromised in the person with diabetes who has developed microvascular changes due to suboptimal diabetes control.

Diabetic cheiroarthropathy or 'stiff joint syndrome' is of particular importance to an anaesthetist, as is may be an indication that the patient is difficult to intubate with an endotracheal tube. The condition is thought to be present in up to 30% of patients with type 1 diabetes and is marked by the presence of a 'positive prayer sign'. With this, patients are unable to achieve contact between their palms and phalangeal joints when the hands are placed together as in prayer.

Postoperative management

During the postoperative phase Julie will require regular measurements for temperature, pulse, respiration and blood pressure recordings, according to local protocol. The aim is to be able to detect early any incidence of haemorrhage, shock or bowel perforation. In addition to the postoperative care that all patients require, Julie is at risk of developing particular diabetes-related complications because of the delicate metabolic balance between insulin and its counter-regulatory hormones. These specific complications will need to be assessed for and treated promptly.

1. Blood transfusion

One such specific concern is related to the infusion of red blood cells. If Julie begins to haemorrhage or loses a significant amount of blood intra- or postoperatively, she may require the rapid infusion of a number of packs of red blood cells.

Key point

Packs of red blood cells contain glucose and therefore may impact on blood glucose levels, causing them to rise and putting the person at risk of hyperglycaemia and ketoacidosis.

During the infusion, should it be required, Julie's blood glucose levels will need to be monitored half-hourly, or according to local procedures, and any hyperglycaemia will need to be corrected quickly and efficiently by increasing the intravenous insulin infusion rate.

2. Blood glucose monitoring

In the general postoperative period, hourly measurements of blood glucose should be recorded routinely in all people with diabetes. This can be via capillary blood and a hand-held blood glucose meter while the results remain generally within the normal parameters. However, should hypo- or hyperglycaemia develop, a venous blood glucose sample may be required as the small, hand-held monitors become less accurate in these situations.

The recording of blood glucose levels hourly requires a great deal of nursing time, which means that it consumes nursing resources and is a costly, but essential, exercise. It is also a repeatedly painful procedure for the patient. An alternative would be to monitor glucose levels via the use of a continuous blood glucose monitoring system. With this, a small transducer is inserted under the patient's skin and the blood glucose levels in the interstitial tissues are recorded every 5 minutes, thus reducing the demand on nursing time and the need to frequently prick the patient's finger. The results can then be seen and a record printed. Unfortunately, while this technology has been developed, it is still costly and is not currently available for widespread monitoring but may become so in the not too distant future.

3. Oxygenation and blood pressure control

Maintenance of adequate oxygenation and blood pressure is important in all patients postoperatively, but even more so in patients with diabetes as these people have higher incidences of cardiac and renal insufficiency. Intravenous fluid administration must be monitored carefully via an accurately completed fluid balance chart to ensure that adequate cardiac output and renal perfusion is maintained. It must be remembered that the presence of glycosuria will induce an osmotic diuresis, leading to inaccuracies in fluid balance measurements. This provides a further rationale for the person's blood glucose levels to remain within the parameters of normal.

4. Fasting

As Julie has undergone bowel surgery, she will need to be fasted until normal bowel function returns and bowel sounds are heard. Even though she is fasting she will still have basal insulin requirements that will need to be met. The insulin, dextrose and potassium sliding-scale regimen will therefore remain *in situ* with the insulin being delivered intravenously according to Julie's hourly blood glucose recordings and the glucose feedback algorithm. Her subcutaneous Lantus® insulin will also continue to be given once-daily at 10 p.m.

5. Sliding-scale insulin infusion

The sliding-scale insulin infusion with dextrose and potassium will be maintained until Julie is able to tolerate oral diet and fluids again. Once this is achieved, the sliding scale can be discontinued and Julie recommenced on her preoperative insulin regimen.

There are some important issues to consider when discontinuing the sliding scale:

1. Once the intravenous insulin has been switched off/disconnected, within 10–15 minutes the person will no longer have any active short-acting insulin in their body unless they are able to make some insulin themselves. If the Lantus® insulin injections have been continued as they should have been, then Julie will not be completely insulin depleted and will have the required basal insulin still circulating in an effective form. She will therefore need to commence her rapid-acting NovoRapid® insulin, which should be given immediately prior to each of her meals or within 15 minutes of eating to avoid hyperglycaemia and potential ketoacidosis.

    For the person with diabetes who has twice-daily injections of mixed insulin, these will have been stopped when the intravenous insulin was commenced. Therefore, prior to stopping and disconnecting the sliding-scale insulin regimen, these particular patients need to be given subcutaneous insulin and this needs to have reached a therapeutic blood value. Once this is achieved – approximately 2 hours after injection – then the intravenous insulin can be discontinued.

2. Owing to the physiological stress of the surgery and the resulting insulin resistance, Julie's daily insulin requirements may need to be increased initially. However, it also needs to be recognized that for some patients who may have had a high calorie intake preoperatively, this will be significantly reduced in the initial postoperative period, thus creating a lower than usual insulin demand. These individual factors need to be considered if optimal glycaemic control is to be achieved in the postoperative period.

    By calculating how many insulin units Julie has received over the preceding 24 hours, including the intravenous insulin and the Lantus® insulin, it would be possible to calculate her initial daily insulin needs fairly accurately. The total number of daily units should then be split thus – 50% basal insulin (Lantus®) and 50% bolus insulin (NovoRapid®), which is further divided between each of the three main meals, taking into account the amount and type of carbohydrate eaten at each meal.

In this scenario, as there is active basal insulin already circulating, it is possible to stop/disconnect the sliding-scale intravenous insulin immediately, as long as the rapid-acting insulin is given with each meal.

3. For patients with diabetes who are treated via a twice-daily subcutaneous mixed insulin such as Mixtard® 30, their total daily insulin requirements can be calculated by simply adding up how much intravenous insulin will have been given over the preceding 24 hours, as no long-acting insulin will have been given in conjunction with this. As a rule of thumb, the total daily insulin dose is then divided into thirds, with two-thirds given in the morning and the remaining third in the evening.

In this instance, as there is no basal insulin, the Mixtard® 30 will need to be given 30–45 minutes before breakfast *and the sliding-scale insulin continued for approximately a further 2 hours*. This will allow the short- and longer-acting insulins contained within the Mixtard® 30 to become active, thus preventing the person from becoming insulin deplete and at risk of hyperglycaemia and ketoacidosis.

It will be possible to identify when the subcutaneous insulin becomes more and more active as the person's intravenous insulin requirements will gradually lessen. It is when this becomes apparent that the sliding-scale insulin regimen can be safely discontinued.

Key point

At no point should the sliding-scale intravenous insulin infusion be discontinued in a person requiring insulin as part of their diabetes treatment without them having been given subcutaneous insulin *and* for this to be in an active state.

In all of the above instances it should be recognized that a person's insulin requirements will change rapidly and frequently as their condition improves and as a result they will need to be reassessed every 2–3 days.

6. Wounds

The development of surgical site infection is a well-known complication of any surgical procedure that damages the integrity of the skin. This may not occur in the immediate postoperative period as studies have shown that most surgical site infections occur within 21 days of surgery and 12–84% are diagnosed once the patient has been discharged home (Mangram *et al.* 1999, cited in Goldrick 2003).

As for all people with a surgical incision site, Julie will require her dressings and any drains to be observed regularly for signs of blockage, haemorrhage or excess discharge, and her temperature recorded at least 4-hourly to observe for pyrexia, which may indicate a wound infection.

Hyperglycaemia plays a key role in the health and healing rate of the wound. It is known that hyperglycaemia inhibits many of the functions of the leucocytes, including impairing phagocytosis, delaying chemotaxis and depressing bacteriocidal capacity, making infection more likely (Hill 2002). It is also known to impair wound healing as it exhibits detrimental effects on the collagen formation process, which results in diminished wound tensile strength (Plodkowski and Edelman 2001).

Conversely, during this period the risks of the person developing a general infection are greater and may include wound, bladder or respiratory tract infections. The presence of any infection will cause blood glucose levels to rise and hyperglycaemia and diabetic ketoacidosis may develop as a result. This therefore needs to be regularly assessed for, and both the infection and hyperglycaemia treated promptly and effectively with appropriate antibiotics and insulin.

During any episode of hyperglycaemia where the blood glucose level rises to ≥15 mmol/l it is necessary to test for ketones in the person's blood or urine. The presence of ketones indicates the development of ketoacidosis which can be life threatening and require emergency treatment (see Chapter 3).

7. Pain and mobility

Two further variables that will affect blood glucose control during the postoperative period are pain and limited mobility due to the pain and surgical incision site. Studies seem to indicate that the analgesic effect of morphine is attenuated in the presence of hyperglycaemia, making people with poorly controlled diabetes experience more pain postoperatively and therefore require larger doses of morphine to achieve effective pain relief (Karci et al. 2004). This indicates a further need for the healthcare team to assess the person's level of pain accurately and to closely monitor for and avoid the development of hyperglycaemia in the postoperative period. The presence of high blood glucose levels should be treated promptly with insulin but it should also be considered that blood glucose levels may fall as the pain relief becomes more effective. In these circumstances, the balance between hyperglycaemia and hypoglycaemia is quite delicate and intricate.

Julie needs to be kept as pain free as possible to minimize the effects of the stress response on blood glucose control, while at the same time recognizing that during this period her insulin requirements will change, potentially quite dramatically. The autonomic stress response to the pain and the lack of mobility will initially increase her daily insulin need.

Effective pain relief will cause the stress response to fall and will enable Julie to become more physically mobile and active. As this happens, she will develop increased sensitivity to the prescribed insulin and her overall, daily insulin requirements may need to be reduced.

On discharge from hospital and for some weeks, despite an excellent recovery, Julie is not going to be as active as she was prior to surgery. The number of insulin units she was taking pre-hospitalization and surgery may no longer be appropriate for her during the time of recovery and healing and as a consequence her total daily insulin dose may need to be increased temporarily. Julie needs to be advised that as she returns to normal eating, drinking and levels of exercise she may identify a need to gradually decrease her insulin doses until her blood glucose levels fall within the range of 4–7 mmol/l preprandially and 2 hours postprandially.

Surgery in different types of diabetes

Day surgery

Day surgery for people with diabetes is no longer contraindicated with modern anaesthetics, surgical procedures and diabetes-monitoring devices; however, the patient must have well-controlled diabetes before day surgery would be considered.

What is not fully known, is the level of metabolic control people with diabetes are able to achieve postoperatively and postdischarge. It therefore seems prudent to make sure that people with diabetes undergoing day surgery are fully aware of the physiological changes that can occur in relation to glycaemic control as a result of surgery. They also need to be adequately prepared and informed to be able to monitor and amend antidiabetes treatments accordingly prior to and following discharge from hospital.

Patients also need to be aware of, and be able to respond to, factors such as the effect of temporary, limited mobility on blood glucose control and to recognize that their food intake may be less initially, thus requiring reduced doses of insulin and/or medication. Patient education covering these lifestyle topics needs to be undertaken to help prevent potential serious repercussions, e.g. the development of hypo- or hyperglycaemia.

The precise actions that need to be taken pre- and postoperatively with regard to antidiabetes medication will depend largely on what medication the person is taking, the length and complexity of the surgery, the time spent nil by mouth and his or her position on the operating list. As mentioned previously, ideally the person with diabetes should be positioned at the top of the theatre list to help avoid potential difficulties and complications.

Tables 5.2 and 5.3 offer guidance on the actions that can be taken relating to the more common antidiabetes treatment modalities. The main aim is to ensure that when the person commences their period of nil by mouth there is little or no active, synthetic insulin that can cause hypoglycaemia. Additionally, insulin produced in excess of demand, e.g. when a person is taking sulphonylureas, also needs to be avoided, again to prevent the occurrence of hypoglycaemia pre- and postoperatively.

Table 5.2 Day surgery in type 1 diabetes.

Treatment	Action preoperative	Action postoperative
Twice daily mixed insulin: • Mixtard® 30 • Novomix® 30 • Humalog® Mix 25 • Humalog® Mix 50 • Humulin® M3	Give insulin as usual the day before surgery. Withhold insulin injection the morning of surgery (Levy 2006). Monitor blood glucose levels hourly. If the person is to be operated on in the afternoon, a percentage of their usual morning dose of insulin may be given with an early, light breakfast. In surgery lasting more than 2 hours or if blood glucose levels rise to >10 mmol/l a sliding-scale insulin infusion will be required.	Recommence insulin injections when eating and drinking is tolerated. Give Mixtard® 30–45 min prior to a main meal. Give with food – *not between meals.* Discontinue sliding-scale insulin regimen as described above. Monitor blood glucose levels 1–2 hourly until stable, then 2 hours postprandial.
Basal/bolus insulin: • Lantus®/Levemir® and Novorapid®/Humalog®/Apidra®	Continue the basal insulin (Lantus/Levemir) at usual time of day and current dose. Patient will need hourly blood glucose monitoring and may require a 5% dextrose infusion to prevent hypoglycaemia. If nil by mouth from midnight, discontinue bolus insulin (Novorapid®/Humalog®) from midnight. If nil by mouth after light breakfast, give 50% of bolus insulin dose with breakfast, then discontinue.	Continue to give basal insulin as same time the patient gives it each day. Recommence bolus insulin when eating resumes. May need to reduce dose to take into account reduced food intake. If hyperglycaemia develops (blood glucose >10 mmol/l) take an additional insulin 'correction dose'. As a rule of thumb, *one unit of insulin will reduce blood glucose level by approximately 2–3 mmol/l.*
Continuous insulin infusion therapy via insulin pump	Continue insulin administration via pump throughout pre-, intra- and postoperative period. Titrate basal rate of insulin according to blood glucose levels recorded half hourly.	—
Tablet therapy in conjunction with insulin therapy	See below	See below

Table 5.3 Day surgery in type 2 diabetes.

Treatment	Action preoperative	Action postoperative
Diet and exercise	No special precautions required if the person's diabetes is well controlled.	Resume healthy diet and exercise regimen when able. Monitor blood glucose levels 2–4 hourly in initial postoperative period.
Short/medium acting sulphonylurea: • Glipizide • Gliclazide	As these newer sulphonlyureas have a much shorter duration of action than previous ones, they can just be withheld on the morning of surgery. Monitor blood glucose levels every 30 min.	Recommence when the person is able to resume normal eating and drinking. Take with next main meal and thereafter as prescribed. Monitor blood glucose levels 1–2 hourly initially and then preprandial and 2 hours postprandial.
Long-acting sulphonylurea: • Glibenclamide • Chlorpropramide	As these drugs have a long action time, they should be stopped 48–72 hours prior to surgery to ensure the majority of the drug has been excreted and is inactive at the time of fasting. This will help to minimize the risk of hypoglycaemia pre- and postoperatively. Monitor blood glucose levels every 30 min.	Recommence the following day if the person is able to tolerate diet and fluids. Take with breakfast and thereafter as prescribed. Monitor blood glucose levels as above.
Metformin	Stopped 48 hours preoperatively to prevent the possibility of lactic acidosis if the person's renal function becomes compromised due to the surgery or its complications.	Recommence as soon as the person is eating and drinking again and the risk of renal impairment has subsided. Take with meals as prescribed.
Thiazolidinedione: • Pioglitazone • Rosiglitazone	Can be continued as they do not cause oversecretion of insulin and have a long duration of action.	If stopped, recommence the morning after surgery and take as prescribed.
Meglitinide: • Repaglinide • Nateglinide	These drugs enhance the secretion of insulin and should be withdrawn when the patient becomes nil by mouth.	Recommence with the next main meal then take as prescribed.
Acarbose	Stop while the person is nil by mouth.	Recommence with the next main meal, then take as prescribed.

Table 5.3 *Continued*

Treatment	Action preoperative	Action postoperative
DPP-4 inhibitor: • Sitagliptin	As these drugs act on the gastrointestinal system and do not increase insulin production, it is safe to continue taking these throughout the pre- and postoperative period. Particularly as the patient will eat again shortly after the operation.	Continue as prescribed.
Incretin mimetic: • Exanatide	As for sitagliptin. Continue as prescribed.	Continue as prescribed.

DPP-4, dipeptidyl peptidase-4.

At the same time healthcare professionals also need to be mindful of the development of hyperglycaemia and potential ketoacidosis. If an intravenous infusion is required and diabetes treatment has been withdrawn preoperatively, then normal saline 0.9% should be the prescribed solution. Intravenous dextrose should be avoided in the absence of insulin or oral medication as there will be no active mechanism to counteract the rise this will cause in blood glucose levels.

Emergency surgery

With emergency surgery it is not always possible to achieve good metabolic control beforehand, particularly if the person's life is dependent on the surgery. In this instance, for the safety and health outcomes of the person any diabetic ketoacidosis would need to be corrected prior to anaesthesia.

All patients with both type 1 and type 2 diabetes requiring emergency surgery would need to be commenced on an intravenous insulin infusion with 5% dextrose fluid being given concurrently. The number of insulin units given intravenously would be dependent upon a sliding-scale algorithm and blood glucose monitoring and treatment would be as per the case study for Julie above.

Conclusion

As mentioned at the beginning of this chapter, people with diabetes have an increased risk of requiring surgery for cardiac complications, but they also develop other conditions requiring surgery in exactly the same way as a person who does not have diabetes. Regardless of the surgical intervention, the presence of diabetes creates additional problems for the person and healthcare team in the pre-, intra- and postoperative phase.

The case study presented above has been devised in such a way that it raises a number of different implications for practice when caring for a person with diabetes undergoing surgery. It has enabled the effects of anaesthesia and surgery on metabolic and blood glucose control to be critically considered, as well as the management options the healthcare professional is faced with when the person with diabetes is kept nil by mouth, stressed and at an increased risk of infection.

Discussion of the case study has included the optimal care and management of the person with diabetes undergoing elective abdominal surgery and evidence-based rationales for practice have been given.

Finally, the chapter has considered the implications of emergency and day surgery for people with type 1 and type 2 diabetes and has given guidance on how these different situations can be managed.

Diabetes in coronary care

Aims of the chapter

This chapter will:

1. Critically discuss the metabolic syndrome with particular emphasis on the aetiology, prevalence, risk factors, diagnosis and treatment.
2. Consider the role of cholesterol and cholesterol metabolism and the targets to be achieved.
3. Explain the coagulation risk factors, such as endothelial dysfunction, platelet hyperactivity and the altered fibrinogen–fibrin response, which occur more frequently in people with diabetes.
4. Discuss in detail the role obesity plays in the development and treatment of the metabolic syndrome.
5. Provide evidence-based rationales for the management of a person with acute cardiovascular disease and type 2 diabetes.

The most common complication of type 2 diabetes is macrovascular, atheroscelerotic disease, which results in a two- to four-fold greater risk of a person with diabetes experiencing a cardiovascular event, compared to those without diabetes. However, the majority of people with diabetes are not aware of their increase risk of cardiovascular disease, which is worrying, particularly as a number of the significant risk factors can be reduced with appropriate diet and lifestyle interventions.

In any cardiovascular event, the presence of diabetes has been associated with a higher mortality rate. Individuals with type 2 diabetes who have experienced a coronary event are up to five times more likely to die than people without diabetes experiencing the same event (Haffner *et al.* 1998). Furthermore, it is estimated that 80% of people with type 2 diabetes will die prematurely (before the age of 65 years) of cardiovascular complications, with female patients with diabetes being at a particularly increased risk of death. With the explosion in the prevalence of type 2 diabetes, and estimations of over 300 million people worldwide being affected by diabetes by 2030 (Wild *et al.* 2004), this will undoubtedly lead to similar increases in the levels of cardiovascular disease and will impact heavily on current healthcare systems, patients and their families.

Within this chapter consideration will be given to the metabolic syndrome formerly known as syndrome X: what it is; who is at risk of developing it; how it is diagnosed; and how it can be treated or prevented. Leading on from this, and linking into the metabolic syndrome, the role of cholesterol and cholesterol metabolism will be considered and healthy lipid targets highlighted.

Coagulation risk factors that develop in diabetes, including endothelial dysfunction, platelet hyperactivity and the fibrinogen–fibrin response, will also be discussed. Central obesity is also a major player in the metabolic syndrome and the development of cardiovascular disease, therefore this will be analysed in detail.

The management of a person with acute cardiovascular disease and type 2 diabetes will be explored and discussed via a case study of a woman with type 2 diabetes who is admitted to a coronary care unit.

While hypertension is a single risk factor in the development and management of cardiovascular disease, having hypertension and diabetes doubles the risk of cardiovascular disease. Hypertension and its management will be briefly addressed in this chapter, but discussed in further detail in Chapter 7.

Metabolic syndrome

The metabolic syndrome is a concept which has been around in medicine and healthcare for over 80 years. During this time it has undergone a number of name changes, including syndrome X, deadly quartet, and insulin resistance syndrome.

Today, the metabolic syndrome is used to describe a 'soup' of established and emerging, interrelated cardiovascular risk factors that occur within a single individual. These risk factors have been shown to have a direct link in the development of atherosclerotic cardiovascular disease. However, as Matfin (2007) points out, there are differences of opinion regarding the very existence of the metabolic syndrome. Academic debate appears to centre on the lack of a universally accepted definition of the condition, and whether there is a need to cluster the rather disparate risk factors under one heading.

Use of the term metabolic syndrome does, however, provide healthcare professionals with a useful template upon which to ensure a full cardiovascular risk assessment is carried out on a person presenting with one or more risk factors. It is also important in helping to identify individuals who have an increased propensity to develop type 2 diabetes and/or cardiovascular disease.

Figure 6.1 illustrates the more common established and evolving cardiovascular risk factors that make up the metabolic syndrome, but these alter slightly depend-

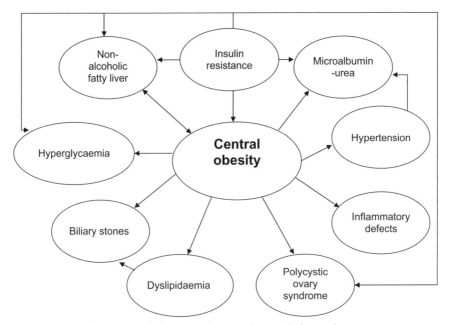

Figure 6.1 Cardiovascular risk factors making up the metabolic syndrome.

ing on which study is followed. Examples of some of the relationships between the risk factors are also indicated here, but this is by no means exhaustive. However, it is commonly accepted that the presence of central obesity causes insulin resistance and has a pivotal role in the development of the metabolic syndrome.

As can be seen in Figure 6.1, the component risk factors of the metabolic syndrome include type 2 diabetes and central obesity. Together, these are two of the most serious public health challenges facing healthcare practitioners all over the world today. Currently, there is no specific treatment for the metabolic syndrome, so individual abnormalities have to be treated as separate entities (Alberti *et al.* 2005).

Diagnosing the metabolic syndrome

Diagnosing the metabolic syndrome is not an easy task due to there not being one clear definition of the condition. Different agencies have developed slightly different measurement criteria, depending on what they consider central to the development of the syndrome. As a consequence, healthcare practitioners across the globe are being encouraged to standardize their assessments by using the measurement tool that has recently been published by the International Diabetes Federation (IDF, 2005). This tool considers central obesity as an essential marker of the metabolic syndrome and builds upon this to include ethnic-specific waist circumference. It is acknowledged by the authors of the tool that while it is simple and easy to use, it will still miss a substantial number of people at risk of the metabolic syndrome as it does not advocate the use of an oral glucose tolerance test to identify individuals with impaired glucose tolerance.

Standardizing metabolic syndrome definitions and measurements can yield positive advances in healthcare, as it will enable comparisons of results from clinical practice to be made and will allow for more accurate estimations of prevalence for instance (Matfin 2007).

According to the new IDF definition, for a person to be diagnosed as having the metabolic syndrome they must have:

- Central obesity – defined as a waist circumference ≥94 cm for Europid men and ≥80 cm for Europid women. These specific values are altered for different ethnic groups identified as being at increased risk.

Individuals must also have *two* of the following four factors:

- Raised triglyceride level (≥1.7 mmol/l) or specific treatment for this lipid abnormality.
- Reduced high-density lipoprotein (HDL) cholesterol (<1.0 mmol/l in males and <1.3 mmol/l in females), or specific treatment for this lipid abnormality.
- Raised blood pressure (systolic ≥130 mmHg or diastolic ≥85 mm/Hg), or treatment of previously diagnosed hypertension.
- Raised fasting plasma glucose (≥5.6 mmol/l) or previously diagnosed type 2 diabetes. If the fasting plasma glucose is >5.6 mmol/l an oral glucose tolerance test is strongly recommended, but it is not necessary to define the presence of the metabolic syndrome (IDF 2005).

Interestingly, the above definition does not take into consideration the 'residual risk factors' of developing cardiovascular disease such as smoking, age, gender and social status. These additional factors could increase a person's risk of cardiovascular disease by as much as 50% (Matfin 2007).

The key components of the metabolic syndrome that have a direct link to type 2 diabetes and its management are discussed in detail below. These include: central obesity, inflammatory defects, dyslipidaemia and hyperglycaemia. As mentioned, hypertension and its management are discussed in greater detail in the next chapter. The mechanics of insulin resistance have been described in detail in Chapter 1.

Central obesity

Obesity is now recognized as one of the major public health concerns in the developing world. It has been shown repeatedly to be associated with the development of heart disease and type 2 diabetes, as well as some cancers. In 2005, 22% of men in England and 24% of women in England were classified as being not just overweight, but obese. By 2050, it is forecast, based upon current trends, that 60% of men and 50% of women in England could be clinically obese (Foresight

2007). Less futuristic figures estimate that in England alone there will be an increase of 2 356 365 obese men and 1 230 573 more obese women in the year 2010 when compared to the 2003 figures (DH 2006). These statistics are clearly worrying and will undoubtedly exert a huge burden on the UK's National Health Service finances and resources.

According to the UK Department of Health (DH 2007), approximately 58% of type 2 diabetes and 21% of heart disease is attributable to excess body fat, and obesity is responsible for approximately 9000 premature deaths under the age of 65 years each year in England alone. Obesity has also been found to reduce life expectancy by an average of 10 years (Donnelly 2005).

Following on from this, people with type 2 diabetes are at a greater risk of developing vascular problems than any other disease-related complication. As a result, cardiovascular complications are the leading cause of death among people with type 2 diabetes, accounting for an estimated 80% of all case fatalities (Donnelly 2005).

There is a strong correlation between obesity and insulin resistance, but it is also acknowledged that some people who are not classed as obese are still insulin resistant and have abnormal levels of metabolic risk factors. These individuals commonly have an abnormal fat distribution that is predominantly situated in the upper body.

This upper-body fat excess can accumulate as visceral fat (intraperitoneally) or as subcutaneous fat. It is the laying down of the visceral fat that has been found to be more closely associated with insulin resistance (Carr *et al.* 2004). Visceral fat releases unusually high levels of non-esterified fatty acids (NEFAs), which contribute to the accumulation of lipids in the liver and muscle as well as adipose tissue (Grundy *et al.* 2005). The oxidation of the lipids in the muscle leads to impairment of insulin-stimulated glucose uptake in the muscle, resulting in higher than normal blood glucose levels.

In addition, the release of the NEFAs also alters hepatic metabolism by increasing the release of glucose from the liver, again resulting in a rise in blood glucose level. In response to this rise, insulin secretion from the beta cells in the pancreas is triggered but the amount of insulin secreted will need to exceed the normal amount, to compensate for the barriers the insulin resistance that is present has created. This results in a state of hyperinsulinaemia, which in turn increases insulin resistance and concludes in a vicious cycle of events.

In the presence of obesity, adipocytes, which are cells that are specialized in storing energy as fat, secrete numerous signalling molecules. Collectively, these molecules are called adipokines and include leptin, adiponectin, tumour necrosis factor α, plasminogen activator inhibitor-1, angiotensin, resistin and interleukin-6.

There is now evidence that tumour necrosis factor α disrupts insulin signalling pathways and desensitizes the insulin receptors on target cells to insulin (Arner 2005). This process occurs because the action of tumour necrosis factor α decreases lipogenesis, increases lipolysis and inhibits the uptake of free fatty acids. This has the net effect of increasing the levels of circulating free fatty acids, which can cause or worsen insulin resistance by impairing insulin signalling pathways further. Tumour necrosis factor α also prevents the recycling of the insulin receptors back on to the surface of the target cells (see Chapter 1). This, in turn, further increases the levels of insulin resistance and ultimately blood glucose levels.

The adipokine adiponectin, on the other hand, is thought to enhance insulin sensitivity in the liver as well as increase fatty acid oxidation and reduce glucose output (Kershaw and Flier 2004). Unfortunately, the levels of adiponectin fall in the presence of obesity; this has a deleterious effect on blood glucose levels as it causes a decrease in insulin sensitivity and fatty acid oxidation and an increase in hepatic glucose output.

Inflammatory defects

The cytokines produced by the adipose tissue cause inflammation and damage to the endothelial layer of the blood vessels. This monolayer of endothelial cells lines the inner aspect of the blood vessels and plays a pivotal role in the regulation of blood flow and nutrient delivery. Hyperglycaemia, hypertension and dyslipidaemia, all found in type 2 diabetes, are thought to contribute to the development of endothelial injury, which is considered to be an early indication of atherosclerosis. It therefore follows that people with poorly controlled type 2 diabetes are at an increased risk of developing potentially fatal atherosclerosis leading to myocardial infarction (MI) or cerebrovascular accident, which subsequently accounts for the high morbidity rate in this group of people.

Endothelial injury also contributes to the development of platelet hyperactivity, which is another common factor in persons with type 2 diabetes. Ordinarily, prostacyclin, which is a prostaglandin, is synthesized and secreted by the endothelial cells to inhibit the activation and aggregation of platelets. Prostacyclin also has a powerful ability to cause vasodilation to help guard against the development of a thrombosis by increasing blood flow. When endothelial dysfunction is present, reduced amounts of prostacyclin are secreted, which causes platelets to become 'stickier' and aggregate more readily. The consequences of this are an increased propensity to thrombus formation and acute MI.

Dyslipidaemia

Lipoproteins transport water-soluble fats around the body via the bloodstream. There are four main types of lipoproteins:

- Chylomicrons and very-low-density lipoprotein (VLDL) which are produced in the gastrointestinal tract and liver respectively and are largely made up of triglycerides.
- Intermediate-density lipoprotein (IDL) formed from remnants of VLDL metabolism.

- Low-density lipoprotein (LDL) formed from the metabolism of IDL
- HDL sourced from the gastrointestinal tract and liver.

In diabetes care, LDL and HDL play significant roles in the development of cardiovascular complications, particularly elevated levels of LDL, as these have been found to correlate very closely with the development of damaging atherosclerosis. Conversely, higher levels of HDL have been identified as offering a protective and preventative effect on the development of atherosclerosis. Therefore in managing the person with diabetes the overall aim should be to decrease levels of circulating LDL and increase the levels of HDL, also known as 'good cholesterol'.

Circulating lipoproteins are generally contained within the blood as the endothelial lining of the blood vessels acts as a barrier, preventing any movement of lipoproteins from the blood. When the endothelium becomes damaged, it allows LDL to pass through the lining and into the intima layer of the vessel wall. Here it undergoes a series of biochemical changes that result in engorgement of the smooth muscle cells in the vessel wall as they fill with cholesterol-rich liquid. This process thus contributes further to the development of atherosclerosis and an increased risk of coronary heart disease (Lilly 2006).

Atherosclerosis

The actual process of atherosclerosis begins with the development of a fatty streak which gradually, over time, builds up to become a fibrous plaque or atheromatus lesion. As a consequence, the vessel wall becomes thick and calcified and a fibrous cap forms causing a narrowing of the lumen which reduces the amount of blood flow along the artery and to the organs that the vessel supplies.

This process renders the blood vessel fragile, more rigid and unable to flex with the normal contraction and relaxation of the artery wall; this makes the endothelium and fibrous cap prone to damage and splitting, creating an even wider area of vessel wall damage. As the fibrous cap splits, it also bleeds, causing a large blood clot to form to seal the damaged area. This blood clot blocks any further blood flow down the damaged artery, and the tissue that the artery supplies becomes infarcted, potentially causing angina pectoris, acute MI and other cardiac disorders, all of which are potentially life threatening.

Hyperglycaemia

In patients with diabetes who have poorly controlled blood glucose levels spanning a period of time, there is a tendency for the hyperglycaemia to cause glycation (adherence of glucose molecules) of the circulating LDL. This confuses the body into thinking that the glycated LDL is a foreign substance and as a result inflammation and antibody production is initiated.

As a result of the hyperglycaemia and inflammatory process, chronic hypersecretion of fibrinogen occurs adversely affecting the blood clotting mechanisms.

Fibrinogen, under the action of thrombin is converted into insoluble fibrin fibres that trap red blood cells, causing the blood to be immobilized into a clot. While this process is usually initiated by tissue damage, it can also occur within an intact blood vessel. It therefore stands to reason that the increase in fibrinogen production increases the person's susceptibility to forming potentially fatal clots within the cardiovascular system.

Case study: Maggie

Maggie is a 51-year-old, white Caucasian woman who works as a receptionist and secretary in a large inner-city high school. She was diagnosed with type 2 diabetes 8 years ago and has always struggled to control her blood glucose levels and reduce her haemoglobin A1c (HbA1c). Over the past 3 years, her HbA1c levels have fluctuated between 8.4 and 9.6% and as a result she has developed peripheral neuropathy in both of her lower legs and feet. Fortunately, she has not, to date, sustained any damage to her feet and limbs and so has not been faced with a slow healing process or the possibility of amputation.

Maggie is also obese with a body mass index (BMI) of 35.1 kg/m². As well as trying endlessly to control her fluctuating blood glucose levels, she has also been trying to lose weight for most of her adult life but finds it very hard. She is able to lose 10–12 kg over a period of time, but finds that she ends up regaining this weight and sometimes more. She does not do any regular form of exercise as she does not like going to the gym, she cannot swim and does not feel safe walking alone in the village in which she lives.

She is married to Tim, who was diagnosed as having a brain tumour a year ago and has been undergoing chemotherapy and radiotherapy. He is currently in a remission period, but Maggie has found dealing with this very stressful, psychologically and emotionally.

Today, while at work, Maggie complains of very severe central chest pain that radiates up to her jaw and down her left arm. She becomes very cold, pale, clammy and short of breath. Her colleagues dial 999 for an ambulance, which arrives within 8 minutes.

The paramedics assess Maggie and administer emergency treatment for an acute MI, including oxygen therapy, 300 mg of oral aspirin and Suscard® 2 mg (buccal tablet) under her lip. Maggie is taken to the nearest hospital and straight into angioplasty for primary percutaneous coronary intervention.

Past medical history

- Type 2 diabetes diagnosed aged 43 years.
- Diabetic neuropathy.

- Dyslipidaemia.
- Hypertension.
- No history of diabetic retinopathy or nephropathy.
- No history of heart disease or stroke.
- Smokes approximately 10–20 cigarettes per day depending on how stressful the day is.

Family history

- Father diagnosed with type 2 diabetes aged 52 years and died of an acute MI aged 69 years.
- Mother still alive but needs medication for hypercholesterolaemia and hypertension.
- Maggie has a younger sister who is alive and well and not diagnosed with diabetes or heart disease. She did, however, have a baby who weighed 4.85 kg at birth.

Medication

- Gliclazide 160 mg twice daily with meals.
- Pioglitazone 30 mg daily.
- Unable to tolerate metformin.

Allergies

- None known.

Examination

- Blood pressure 90/60 mmHg.
- Pulse 98 bpm, regular.
- Temperature 37.4°C.
- Respirations 20/minute.
- Oxygen saturation 94%.
- Random capillary blood glucose level 13.2 mmol/l.
- 12-lead ECG – ST elevation in leads V1, V2, V3, V4 and V5, Q waves in II, III and AVF.
- HbA1c 9.4%.
- Weight 90.1 kg.
- BMI 35.1 kg/m^2.
- Total cholesterol 5.9 mmol/l.
- HDL 0.9 mmol/l.
- LDL 3.4 mmol/l.
- Triglycerides 4.4 mmol/l.

Discussion of Maggie's case

This discussion will look specifically at the care and management Maggie will require during her admission to hospital in relation to her diabetes and how this impacts on clinical outcomes. The MI-specific interventions such as thrombolysis, serial electrocardiograms, etc. will not be considered here.

1. Pathophysiological events during MI

As a consequence of an abruptly occluded coronary vessel, which may occur as a result of atherosclerosis or a thrombus, oxygen levels fall in the myocardium. Ordinarily, the myocardium receives oxygen, which it uses to oxidize NEFAs; however, when the oxygen supply is diminished as is the case in acute MI, the cardiac mitochondria start using glucose for energy as they can metabolize this anaerobically. Detrimentally, this leads to a build-up of lactic acid and causes a lowered blood pH (Lilly 2006).

At the same time, the 'stress response' during MI increases the release of catecholamines, glucagon and cortisol, which increase blood glucose levels and cause or increase existing insulin resistance. People with diabetes are more sensitive to catecholamine stimulation, which causes a dramatic increase in the levels of circulating free fatty acids. The body's response to this is for the myocardium to metabolize free fatty acids as priority over glucose to reduce the overall levels, but this has deleterious effects during MI.

The shift from anaerobic glucose metabolism to aerobic free fatty acid metabolism increases the oxygen demand of the heart muscle. The increased demand cannot be met by the blood supply due to the infarction process. This imbalance in the oxygen supply and demand process creates an energy deficit that is believed to potentiate the damage to the ischaemic myocardium (Cummings *et al.* 1999; Walker 1999).

Myocardial hypoxia also causes a rapid reduction in the intracellular supply of adenosine triphosphate (ATP) which results in: (1) an increase in extracellular potassium, causing potentially fatal arrhythmias; (2) increased intracellular sodium levels, which contribute to cellular oedema; and (3) intracellular calcium accumulating in the myocardial cells, which is thought to exacerbate cell destruction. Collectively, these pathophysiological events decrease myocardial function as early as 2 minutes following the occlusion (Lilly 2006).

2. Role of insulin

Based upon the above, one of the aims of treatment in the acute phase of the MI would be to create an environment in which the myocardium continues to utilize glucose anaerobically rather than the free fatty acids, in an attempt to reduce the overall oxygen demand.

Insulin, either endogenous or exogenous, has been found to prefer the use of glucose over free fatty acids as an energy source. Studies have also shown that insulin may have a role in restoring other cardiac and metabolic dysfunctions that are common in people with diabetes and mentioned earlier. Insulin has been shown to decrease platelet aggregation and normalize the fibrinolytic response; both are important factors in achieving myocardial damage limitation (Cummings *et al.* 1999).

In commencing insulin therapy, numerous studies have looked at the efficiency of this treatment and following a meta-analysis of relevant randomized controlled trials, Pittas *et al.* (2004) concluded that insulin therapy alone was not enough to reduce mortality rates, but had to be used in combination with glycaemic control. The Diabetes Mellitus Insulin Glucose Infusion in Acute Myocardial Infarction (DIGAMI) study (Malmberg *et al.* 1997) aimed to keep blood glucose levels between 7.0 and 10.9 mmol/l following acute MI. In a follow-up study, DIGAMI 2, which was designed to assess the impact of tight blood glucose control, Malmberg *et al.* (2005) randomized patients admitted with acute MI and diabetes into three groups. The first group received a glucose, insulin, potassium (GIK) infusion for 24 hours and blood glucose levels were to be kept between 5 and 7 mmol/l. The second group received the same GIK infusion, but blood glucose targets were not set and the third group did not receive the GIK infusion and were treated as per routine protocol.

While this appeared to be a robust and appropriate piece of research, several unanticipated problems developed, a main one being that the recommended blood glucose targets in the first group were never achieved. All three groups achieved an average blood glucose level of 8.5 mmol/l. Despite this, the study was able to demonstrate that the more severe the hyperglycaemia, the higher the risk of the person developing an adverse outcome (Van den Berghe 2005). This is an important point to consider when managing the care of a person admitted with an acute MI who also has diabetes.

For these reasons, it is now common practice to commence all patients who are admitted with an acute MI and a blood glucose level of ≥11.1 mmol/l on an insulin, dextrose and potassium sliding-scale regimen, regardless of whether they are known to have diabetes or not. This should commence as soon as a diagnosis of suspected MI is made. This practice would apply to Maggie as she has diabetes that will typically be more difficult to control in the acute phase due to the hormonal 'stress response', which acts to increase blood glucose levels and decrease insulin sensitivity. Regardless, she also has a blood glucose level over the threshold.

There does not appear to be a consensus in the literature as to what constitutes an optimal blood glucose level to aim for in order to reduce mortality and morbidity rates. Van den Berghe *et al.* (2001) demonstrated that if blood glucose levels could be stabilized between 4.4 and 6.1 mmol/l, this will have a significant impact on lowering mortality and hospital mortality rates. This is a narrow and potentially difficult target to achieve, therefore it would be reasonable to suggest that if blood glucose levels could be kept within the normal range of 4–7 mmol/l this would have a positive effect on clinical outcomes.

The management of a person on a sliding-scale insulin regimen is described in detail in Chapter 5; however, there are issues pertinent to Maggie which need highlighting.

First, it is imperative that the insulin is not given without a concurrent intravenous dextrose infusion running so as to prevent the development of hypoglycaemia, which would exacerbate the current stress response. As Maggie is showing signs of some left ventricular failure, an infusion of 10% dextrose would be more appropriate than 5% dextrose, to reduce the amount of intravenous fluids she would require. She would require blood glucose monitoring as frequently as necessary to ensure that her blood glucose levels are kept below 10 mmol/l but also avoiding hypoglycaemia.

Careful and regular assessment of her potassium levels would also be required as she is at risk of hypokalaemia due to the decrease in ATP caused by the MI. This risk is increased with the commencement of insulin therapy, which lowers intracellular potassium levels even further (see Chapter 5), thus increasing the risk of Maggie developing cardiac arrhythmias. Potassium should be added to the dextrose infusion in order to maintain Maggie's potassium levels between 4.0 and 5.0 mmol/l and should be given via a controlled drip counter to prevent rapid infusion and overdose.

While Maggie is receiving intravenous insulin she will need to discontinue her pioglitazone, as this is not licensed for use with insulin and is contraindicated with cardiac insufficiency. The gliclazide could also be discontinued as her blood glucose levels are being maintained by the insulin infusion.

The decision of when to discontinue the insulin therapy is a matter for debate. In reviewing the literature, Pittas *et al.* (2004) found that on average, intravenous, sliding-scale insulin was administered for 24–72 hours, but an abnormal blood glucose can persist in vulnerable patients for up to 3 months after the cardiac event. For this reason, some cardiologists/diabetologists continue the insulin therapy beyond the sliding scale for a further 3 months, but this is dependent on the patient being willing and compliant. For someone who does not have diabetes and is admitted to hospital for something that they see as being entirely different, they may have difficulties in commencing a demanding subcutaneous insulin regimen. The education that the person will need is significant if the insulin is to be taken safely and used to control blood glucose levels.

In Maggie's case, as she has been having difficulty maintaining her blood glucose levels over recent months and this has manifested itself as a MI, it would seem sensible for her to commence insulin therapy for a minimum of 3 months. After this period, as she has previously been diagnosed with diabetes, she may need to remain on insulin to control her diabetes. In order to give the best possible chance of controlling blood glucose levels within the normal range of 4–7 mmol/l, Maggie will be commenced on a four injections per day basal/bolus regimen. This will require her to inject a rapid-acting insulin prior to each of her main meals to meet her postprandial high blood glucose levels. She will also need a long-acting, peakless insulin, which she will inject once per day to provide her with her basal insulin requirements.

Maggie will require help, support and education related to the insulin therapy including:

- The action of the different insulins.
- Recognizing and treating hypoglycaemia.
- Injection technique.
- Rotating injection sites.
- Storage of insulin.
- Driving and informing the UK Driver Vehicle Licensing Agency (DVLA).
- Matching carbohydrate intake with insulin requirements.
- Blood glucose monitoring.
- Factors that affect insulin absorption and action, i.e. exercise, hot baths, etc.

3. MI in premenopausal women with type 2 diabetes

In the general population, one of the highest risk factors in the development of MI is being male and middle aged. The incidence of acute MI in younger, middle-aged women is much lower than their equivalent male counterparts. The reason for this is thought to be due to the cardioprotective effect of the female hormones in premenopausal women.

In type 2 diabetes, premenopausal women lose their protection against macrovascular disease and therefore the incidence of MI and stroke in this group is much greater when compared to the general female population who do not have type 2 diabetes (Marshall and Flyvbjerg 2006). The concept of more women developing cardiovascular disease is an evolving one and runs parallel to the increasing numbers of people developing early-onset (under the age of 40 years) type 2 diabetes due to the rising incidence of obesity.

The cardioprotective effect in premenopausal women has been largely taken for granted in medicine and healthcare, resulting in female patients being less likely to be screened and treated for cardiovascular disease. This may also be coupled with concerns about pregnancy and the risk of adverse fetal outcomes with statin and antihypertensive therapy (Song and Hardisty 2007). These traditional views now need to be challenged and practices put into place to ensure that the increased risk of cardiovascular disease in premenopausal women with type 2 diabetes is not only recognized, but effectively treated.

4. Peripheral arterial disease

In addition to highlighting the importance of appropriate care for women, emphasis also needs to be placed on the role of peripheral arterial disease as a precursor to cardiovascular disease. People with peripheral arterial disease are six times more likely to die from cardiovascular disease within 10 years than people without peripheral arterial disease (Belch *et al.* 2007). The incidence increases markedly with age, affecting 3% of people under the age of 60 years, rising to over 20% of people aged over 75 years. Unless specifically screened for, the condition can often go undiagnosed, as around 60% of people with peripheral arterial disease are asymptomatic (Belch *et al.* 2007). This means that patients do not get the proper care until the associated heart disease becomes apparent. It therefore seems appropriate to ensure that people with a high propensity to developing the condition are routinely screened for the presence of peripheral arterial disease and preventative advice and support in helping to eliminate or modify the risk factors is offered on an individual basis.

Maggie has not previously been diagnosed with peripheral arterial disease but she does exhibit a number of the high risk factors associated with this and cardiovascular disease. These include: (i) being overweight/obese; (2) requiring treatment for hypertension; (3) presence of dyslipidaemia; (4) hyperglycaemia related to poorly controlled type 2 diabetes; and (5) being a smoker. The management of these is now discussed in more detail.

5. Obesity management

Achieving and maintaining a healthy body weight (BMI 18–24 kg/m²) is a real challenge to the healthcare practitioners of today and is reflected in Maggie's acknowledgement of her weight problem, which she finds very difficult to rectify.

Maggie openly admits that she does not do any form of regular, planned exercise, yet studies have shown physical activity has a beneficial effect on insulin sensitivity and therefore glucose metabolism. Unfortunately, the positive effects of exercise are short-lasting, meaning that regular exercise is required to sustain the benefits (Astrup 2003).

Significant diet and lifestyle changes are often needed to enable people to lose weight and achieve a level of physical fitness that is beneficial in reducing the risk of developing cardiovascular disease and type 2 diabetes. In the majority of cases, these diet and lifestyle changes involve breaking habits that have built up during a lifetime, and the expectation that the person can change them forever in a very short time only leads to frustration, lack of motivation and failure, for both the patient and the healthcare professional. Realistic weight loss and lifestyle management goals therefore need to be set with Maggie and these should be frequently reviewed.

For anyone who is overweight or obese, the task to achieve satisfactory weight management is far from simple or easy and is compounded by the fact that the current UK National Health Services' approach to obesity management is patchy (Deville-Almond 2003). Much research has shown that if a person is able to lose just 10% of their body weight this corresponds to a reduction in HbA1c level, a lowering of cholesterol levels and a fall in systolic blood pressure (Norris *et al.* 2004). This is certainly achievable with the right advice and support; however, in order to fall within the 'healthy weight range', many people need to lose significantly more than 10% of their body weight. Once the magical 10% is lost, it is crucial that healthcare intervention is continued to keep the person on track and to maintain and build on their excellent weight loss achievement.

Any weight loss, no matter how small or large, has to be maintained over a long period of time in order for the health benefits to be reaped (Norris *et al.* 2004). Maggie acknowledges that for her this is proving to be a challenge, and indeed many people find it difficult to maintain healthy changes in diet and physical activity in the long term (National Heart Lung and Blood Institute 1998). Studies have shown that the majority of obese persons regain most of their lost weight over a 12-month period (Norris *et al.* 2004).

Effective weight loss and management is not just about diet and exercise, it also requires an understanding of all the biological and behavioural factors that have led the patient to become overweight or obese. These include an assessment of any underlying medical problems such as underactive thyroid function, which would contribute to weight gain and would need to be treated in the first instance. The patient's current eating habits and dietary knowledge, their levels of self-esteem and potential motivation, and use of any medications known to cause weight gain also need to be ascertained.

In Maggie's case she is currently taking gliclazide and pioglitazone to help control her blood glucose levels, and these have the known side-effects of weight gain (Bailey and Feher 2004).

Diet

The goals for weight loss should be set, and agreed by Maggie, and should include a target of no further weight gain and a realistic weight loss. It is appropriate to initially aim for a loss of 5–10% of body weight, by reducing weight by 0.5–1 kg per week. All objectives should be recorded and their achievement documented; this can act as a powerful motivation tool for the patient and indeed the healthcare practitioner.

Maggie could be referred to a dietitian for a safe and effective weight loss dietary programme. Additionally, as she also has type 2 diabetes, the glycaemic index (GI) diet described in Chapter 1 would be an excellent starting point as adherence to this would enable weight loss and blood glucose control to be achieved.

In addition to a low GI carbohydrate intake, it is also recommended that fat intake should be confined to the use of monosaturated fats, which are found in nuts, seeds and olives. Lovejoy (2002, cited in Colombani 2004) reported that a diet high in saturated fatty acids, which are generally solid at room temperature and derived from animal sources, can have adverse effects on insulin sensitivity.

Exercise

When diet is coupled with a weight loss exercise programme, the amount of fat lost is greater than when just a dietary programme is followed (Astrup 2003). The current UK government recommendation of exercising 20–30 minutes per day for a minimum of 5 days per week has been shown to be very effective in decreasing insulin resistance (Evans *et al.* 2004). However, it is unlikely that this level of exercise will contribute towards significant weight loss. To gain maximum benefit from exercise, Maggie should ideally undertake at least three exercise sessions per week, each lasting a minimum of 30 minutes and being of moderate to high intensity (Astrup 2003). The planned and regular exercise should cause a 40–60% rise in resting heart rate if weight loss is to be enhanced.

6. Hypertension

High blood pressure, classified as being ≥160/100 mmHg, is on its own a single risk factor in the development of cardiovascular disease and people with diabetes are twice as likely to have raised blood pressure than those without diabetes. Furthermore, people who have diabetes and uncontrolled hypertension double their risk of cardiovascular disease.

The news is not all bad, as according to the UK Perspective Diabetes Study (UKPDS) (1998), a 44% reduction in stroke and an incredible 56% reduction of heart failure can be achieved by achieving tight blood pressure control. The current recommendation by the British Hypertension Society is for people with type 2 diabetes to maintain their blood pressure no higher than 130/80 mmHg to reduce their cardiovascular risk (Williams *et al.* 2004).

In the context of cardiovascular disease, the presence of hypertension can have devastating effects. It will increase the workload of the heart and cause damage to the arterial and venous walls, including hypertrophy of the smooth muscle layer, and exacerbate endothelial cell dysfunction and cause fatigue of the elastic fibres in the arterial and venous walls. As mentioned earlier, disruption of the endothelial lining in the blood vessels promotes the development of damaging and potentially fatal atherosclerosis. In the presence of hypertension, atherosclerosis develops even more rapidly (Lilly 2006).

Lifestyle measures to lower blood

Lifestyle modification has been found to be effective in lowering blood pressure in people who are not taking any antihypertensive medication and also in those who are being treated pharmacologically. Regardless of the need for tablet therapy, lifestyle advice should be initiated at diagnosis.

The interventions shown in Table 6.1 have been shown to have a positive effect on lowering a person's blood pressure, but they need to be continued once the blood pressure has returned to within an acceptable range (Williams *et al.* 2004). It can be seen that by adopting simple lifestyle measures the person with hypertension can reduce his or her systolic blood pressure by 23–45 mmHg. This could be enough to limit the need to commence antihypertensive medication.

However, in the person with diabetes, if lifestyle measures are not sufficiently effective, or the person has a sustained systolic blood pressure between 140 and 159 mmHg or a diastolic blood pressure between 90 and 99 mmHg, then pharmacological treatment would be indicated.

Antihypertensive drug therapy

Currently, there are more than 100 drug preparations designed to treat hypertension, but in the person with diabetes an angiotensin-converting enzyme (ACE) inhibitor would be the first drug of choice as it has additional benefits over and above lowering blood pressure. It reduces blood pressure by blocking the conversion of angiotensin I to angiotensin II, which in turn limits vasoconstriction, reduces sodium retention and decreases sympathetic nervous system activity. It also increases the amount of circulating bradykinin, which causes vasodilation.

Table 6.1 Lifestyle strategies to reduce blood pressure levels (Williams *et al.* 2004).

Recommendation	Expected systolic blood pressure reduction
Achieve and maintain a 'healthy' body mass index of 20–24.4 kg/m²	5–10 mmHg per 10 kg weight loss
Ensure a diet that is rich in fruit, vegetables, low-fat diary products and an overall reduction of saturated and total fat intake	8–14 mmHg
Limit the amount of dietary sodium to <100 mmol/day (<2.4 g sodium or <6 g sodium chloride) NB: Food labels list levels of sodium chloride, this needs to be multiplied by 2.5 to gain the sodium content	2–8 mmHg
Commit to regular aerobic physical activity, e.g. brisk walking for at least 30 min on most days of the week	6–9 mmHg
Limit alcohol consumption to: • Men ≤21 units/week • Women ≤14 units/week	2–4 mmHg

It must be recognized that achieving the target level for blood pressure in some people is quite difficult. These people may require a 'cocktail' of different anti-hypertensive drugs to ensure that their blood pressure is kept at or below 130/80 mmHg. This can be problematic due to the increased risk of side-effects as more drugs are prescribed and the likely difficulties relating to compliance and polypharmacy.

7. Dyslipidaemia

The Heart Protection Study Collaborative Group (2002) reported that the use of statin therapy can reduce the incidence of cardiovascular events and death by 25% in high-risk patients with type 2 diabetes. The results of this study are equally applicable to those people who have type 2 diabetes and cardiovascular disease, as well as those whose coronary heart disease risk is 15% or more over 10 years, but do not have type 2 diabetes.

In prescribing medication to reduce dyslipidaemia in diabetes, Grundy *et al.* (2005) postulates that reducing the level of LDL in the blood should be the primary target for therapy. Once this has been achieved, then the focus can turn to increasing the HDLs and reducing the levels of circulating triglycerides. Patients with type 2 diabetes do not generally have particularly elevated LDL concentrations, instead they typically have elevated triglyceride and reduced HDL levels and small, dense LDL particles. Currently, there are not sufficient data to provide guidance on how these blood anomalies can be best treated.

The two main cholesterol-lowering drugs (statins) prescribed are simvastatin and atorvastatin. Indeed simvastatin 10 mg can now be obtained over the counter in a pharmacy without prescription. In some respects this may provide some cardiovascular benefit to the people who buy and take it regularly, but the Heart Protection Study Collaboration Group (2002) report that 40 mg of simvastatin needs to be taken daily for it to be beneficial. Therefore 10 g daily is only one-quarter of the recommended dose.

Additionally, buying over-the-counter statins could be detrimental if the person's mindset is programmed to think 'take the tablet, eat what I like' (e.g. a high fat diet). There is also the argument that over-the-counter statins will only be bought by the people who care about their lipid levels and are therefore probably already following a healthy diet – a case of 'preaching to the converted'.

Treating patients with simvastatin 40 mg daily has been shown to reduce LDL by approximately 1.0 mmol/l, which equates to a significant 22% reduction in the first-event incidence of a major coronary event, stroke or revascularization and this is the drug of choice according to the Heart Protection Study Collaboration Group (2002).

However, the Collaborative Atorvastatin Diabetes Study (CARDS) provides robust evidence for the use of atorvastatin 10 mg daily as a primary prevention against major cardiovascular events in patients with type 2 diabetes (Colhoun *et al.* 2004). This study found that coronary heart events were reduced by an impressive 36% in people who had type 2 diabetes and took atorvastatin 10 mg daily.

The evidence on the use of statin therapy in the reduction of cardiovascular events is so convincing that the Joint British Societies (JBS) have produced guidelines recommending statin use in all patients with both type 1 and type 2 diabetes aged over 40 years, irrespective of their cholesterol levels (JBS 2005).

Maggie is not currently prescribed any lipid-lowering drugs, yet her cholesterol and triglyceride levels on admission are out of the target ranges. With the history of now two cardiovascular events, Maggie is a prime candidate to commence statin therapy. As the cardiovascular outcomes are slightly better, atorvastatin 10 mg daily could be the drug of choice.

In considering a number of different relevant and credible research studies, Erdmann (2007) explored the role of the thiazolidinediones (TZDs), pioglitazone and rosiglitazone, in lipid metabolism. He reported that similar to statins, TZDs seemed to have a number of different metabolic effects that appeared to positively influence cardiovascular outcomes.

Although there are currently few studies that directly investigate the metabolic effects of a TZD when added to statin therapy, Erdmann (2007) reports that when pioglitazone was added to existing statin therapy in a patient with considerable lipid abnormalities, significant improvements in total cholesterol, HDL and triglycerides were seen. Similarly, rosiglitazone has been found to increase LDL buoyancy and particle size and decrease small dense LDL levels when added to statin therapy. Erdmann (2007) also reports that rosiglitazone can be beneficial in reducing blood pressure in patients with type 2 diabetes receiving statin therapy.

It therefore appears that the introduction of TZDs in addition to statin therapy may improve the clinical outcomes for patients with type 2 diabetes and dyslipidaemia. Indeed, with Maggie already taking pioglitazone, the introduction of a statin to reduce lipid levels could have greater benefits than anticipated. However, this could only be a treatment option if she were to discontinue the prescribed insulin therapy. Further clinical trials looking into this issue are awaited with anticipation.

8. Hyperglycaemia

Today, it is widely recognized that improving glycaemic control to achieve an HbA1c of <7% reduces the incidence and severity of microvascular complications; however, it may also have a role in decreasing the risk of macrovascular disease (American Diabetes Association 2005b).

For many years now, metformin has been thought to have protective vascular properties. Experimental and clinical trials have demonstrated that metformin helps to prevent the development of atherosclerosis, improves endothelial dysfunction and exerts antifibrinolytic effects, thus reducing the incidence of intravascular clotting (Wiernsperger 2007). It has also been shown to increase cardiac blood flow by up to 40% 6 months after treatment for ischaemia, and has a protective effect on the heart during the post-ischaemic phase (Wiernsperger 2007). It therefore appears prudent, at the time of diagnosis, to commence all patients with type 2 diabetes on metformin for its cardioprotective properties, regardless of their blood glucose and HbA1c levels.

'Metabolic memory' is a new and emerging concept within the field of diabetes care and management. Ihnat et al. (2007) describe this phenomenon as the presence of postprandial hyperglycaemia in the early stages of the disease process leaving an imprint on cells. This imprint 'programmes' the cells to become dysfunctional, leading to the development of future cardiovascular complications. This therefore highlights the need for early and aggressive glycaemic management and control.

Furthermore, data from the Epidemiology of Diabetes Interventions and Complications (EDIC) trial and the UKPDS (Ihnat et al. 2007) strengthen the case further for good glycaemic control from the time of diagnosis. Both trials suggest that people with lower fasting blood glucose levels at the time of diagnosis have fewer vascular complications and fewer adverse clinical outcomes when compared to people with higher blood glucose levels. Metformin and pioglitazone have been found to exert positive benefits both in reducing blood glucose levels and preventing vascular damage.

Antiplatelet therapy with aspirin 75 mg daily is also a beneficial therapeutic intervention post-cardiovascular event, due to its antithrombotic properties. Some physicians choose to commence aspirin 75 mg as a prophylactic measure in patients with type 2 diabetes and therefore at increased risk of cardiovascular disease. However, currently there is no evidence to support the use of aspirin as a primary preventative drug and caution must be taken in prescribing aspirin over long periods of time.

General care and management

In addition to the above specific management and care of the person with diabetes experiencing a cardiovascular event, there are a number of more generic actions that need to be taken to help prevent further, potentially deleterious, cardiovascular incidents.

The National Institute for Health and Clinical Excellence (NICE 2008) provides clear guidance for the assessment and management of cardiovascular risk in patients with type 2 diabetes. For those people who are perceived to be at a high premature cardiovascular risk for their age, NICE (2008) recommends estimating a person's individual cardiovascular risk annually using the UK Prospective Diabetes Study risk engine (see http://www.dtu.ox.ac.uk/index.php?maindoc=/riskengine/) and to use this risk assessment as an educational tool when discussing the results with the person. NICE (2008) also suggests that a full lipid profile should be undertaken when assessing cardiovascular risk after diagnosis of type 2 diabetes and before commencing lipid-modifying therapy.

Conclusion

As mentioned at the beginning of this chapter, macrovascular and atherosclerotic disease is the most common complication of type 2 diabetes. The presence of the metabolic syndrome has a significant role to play in the development of diabetic macrovascular disease and this chapter has highlighted and discussed the aetiology, prevalence and risk factors of the metabolic syndrome. Diagnosis and treatment have also been considered, with emphasis on the role of cholesterol and cholesterol metabolism and the ideal targets that need to be achieved to reduce the risk of cardiovascular disease and morbidity.

Coagulation risk factors have also been addressed and the case study represents a typical presentation of a person with acute MI secondary to diabetes. Within the case study, issues such as insulin treatment, obesity, hormonal response and general management and treatment have been considered, with evidence-based rationales provided to underpin the discussion.

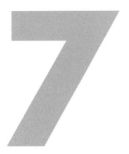

Management of diabetes in the renal unit

Aims of the chapter

This chapter will:

1. Outline the structure of the kidney, and explain the renal physiology.
2. Discuss how changes in the structure and function of the kidney, due to poorly controlled diabetes, result in the development of diabetic nephropathy.
3. Identify the stages of diabetic nephropathy, the criteria to aid diagnosis and the need for effective screening.
4. Critically analyse and discuss the management of a person with type 2 diabetes who has developed end-stage renal disease.
5. Offer suggestions on how the development of diabetic nephropathy can be either prevented or delayed.

Diabetic nephropathy is a common, serious and costly complication of diabetes. It is found to develop in 30–50% of people with type 1 diabetes and up to 25% of people with type 2 diabetes. It is the most common cause of all case, end-stage renal disease, and is thought to account for a massive 39% of the total healthcare costs for diabetes (Happich *et al.* 2008).

This chapter outlines the pathophysiology, incidence and diagnosis of diabetic nephropathy and considers the evidence from the United Kingdom Prospective Diabetes Study (UKPDS) (Stratton *et al.* 2000) and the Diabetes Control and Complications Trial (Diabetes Control and Complications Research Group 1995) for the need to achieve good glycaemic control in order to reduce the incidence of diabetic nephropathy.

The management of diabetic nephropathy is discussed via a case study of a person with long-standing, poorly controlled diabetes who has been admitted to hospital for haemodialysis. Continuous ambulatory peritoneal dialysis will not be discussed, as this tends to be dealt with on an out-patient basis.

Anatomy and physiology of the normal functioning kidney

In health, there are two kidneys located on either side of the vertebral column, which are served by the renal artery and renal vein (Figure 7.1). These enter and exit the kidney at a prominent indentation called the hilus. The renal cortex is the outer layer of the kidney and is covered on its outer aspect by the fibrous renal capsule. Renal medulla sit within the cortex and are made up of approximately 6–18 triangular or conical structures called renal pyramids. The bases of the pyramids face the cortex and the tips project into the renal sinus. The tips of the renal pyramids are called renal papilla and they drain urine into the minor calyx, which is a cup-shaped structure. Four or five minor calyx merge to create a major calyx. The major calyx then continues to merge further to form the renal pelvis, which is connected to the ureter along which urine is drained and collected in the bladder (Martini and Kareleskint 1998).

The kidney has a major role to play in a number of different bodily mechanisms, including the excretion of water and solutes such as sodium, potassium and hydrogen. This is carefully regulated by the proximal tubule, loop of Henle and the distal convoluted tubule. These structures sit partly in the cortex and partly in the medulla of the kidney.

The kidney is also responsible for excreting some of the waste products of metabolism such as urea, creatinine and uric acid, in order to create the stable

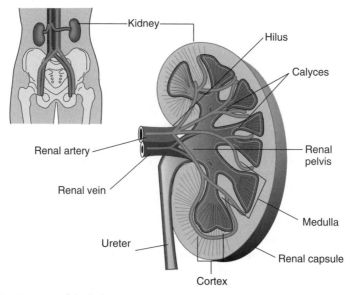

Figure 7.1   Structure of the kidney.

extracellular environment that is necessary for cells to be able to function effectively.

In contrast to the kidney's excretory role, renin, angiotensin II and prostaglandins are produced by the kidney to regulate the systemic and renal haemodynamics. In addition, erythropoietin is secreted as part of normal red blood cell production and calcitriol, a metabolite of vitamin D, is also secreted by the kidney in its role to maintain mineral metabolism (Rennke and Denker 2007).

The normal, healthy kidney will filter approximately 120–145 litres of blood per day in women and 165–180 litres/day in men. The amount of blood filtered is termed the glomerular filtration rate (GFR) and gives an indication of the level of functioning in the kidney; however, the GFR starts to decline by 10 ml per decade from the age of 30 years as part of the normal ageing process. Therefore, a person who is generally fit and well in their 70s may have a GFR of only 90 litres/day.

The final stages of glomerular filtration are witnessed in the production of urine, which should be a clear, straw-coloured fluid.

Figure 7.2 shows the structure of a normal renal tubule and its associated blood supply. This is simply a long tubular passageway that is subdivided into different regions, all having different structural and functional characteristics. It is estimated that there are approximately 1.25 million renal tubules in each kidney (Martini and Karleskint 1998).

Blood initially enters the glomerulus. This is a capillary knot situated in the Bowman's capsule, within the renal cortex. Blood arrives at the glomerulus via the afferent arteriole and leaves by the efferent arteriole. Filtrate forms at the glomerulus

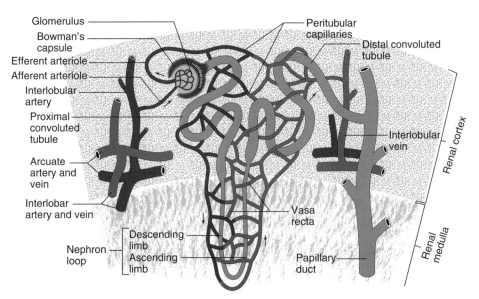

Figure 7.2 Renal tubule.

as blood pressure forces fluid and dissolved solutes out of the glomerular capillaries and into the cup-shaped Bowman's capsule. This process produces a protein-free solution that is very similar to blood plasma and is known as filtrate.

During the process of filtration, solutes are able to pass across a barrier depending on the size of the solute and the size of the pores in the filter. In the kidney, the pores of the filter need to be large enough to allow organic waste products to pass through to enable them to be excreted, but a consequence of this is that water, ions and smaller, useful molecules such as glucose, fatty acids and amino acids also pass through the filter as they are smaller. The kidney is therefore structured in such a way to enable these useful and required substances to be reclaimed.

From the Bowman's capsule, the filtrate enters the proximal convoluted tubule, which is lined by simple cuboidal epithelium with a microvillous surface. Here water, ions, including potassium and sodium, and all other organic nutrients such as glucose are selectively reabsorbed and released into the peritubular fluid that surrounds the renal tubule (Martini and Karleskint 1998). At the same time, creatinine, antibiotics, diuretics and uric acid are secreted into the lumen of the proximal convoluted tubule ready for excretion.

The proximal convoluted tubule ends at the descending limb of the loop of Henle, which takes the fluid through the medulla of the kidney towards the renal pelvis. The ascending limb of the loop of Henle returns the fluid towards the cortex. As fluid passes through the loop of Henle, active transport mechanisms 'pump' water, sodium, potassium, magnesium and calcium out of the tubule, resulting in 35–40% of the filtered sodium and chloride being reabsorbed. This process results in an unusually high concentration of solutes in the tubule fluid at this point.

The loop of Henle connects to the distal convoluted tubule, which is an important site for the selective reabsorption of further water, sodium, chloride and calcium from the tubular fluid, while at the same time enabling the secretion of potassium, hydrogen and urea.

Each renal tubule empties into a collecting tubule, which transports the fluid to a collecting duct. The collecting duct receives tubular fluid from a number of different tubules and eventually drains into a minor calyx. Selective reabsorption and secretion continues in the collecting ducts, which are now under hormonal control. Sodium levels are controlled by aldosterone, which increases the levels of sodium reabsorption, and atrial natriuretic peptide, which decreases the amount of sodium to be reabsorbed.

Under basal conditions, the collecting tubules are relatively impermeable to water unless they are exposed to antidiuretic hormone released from the posterior pituitary gland. As the body becomes dehydrated, levels of circulating antidiuretic hormone will increase, causing additional water to filter out of the distal convoluted tubule and collecting duct and return to the body where it is needed. This has the effect of causing the urine to become more concentrated and darker in colour. If less fluid is required by the body, the levels of antidiuretic hormone decline, allowing the water to remain in the collecting ducts and be excreted. The urine therefore becomes more dilute as a result of this process. If the kidneys were not able to perform the function of concentrating the urine, fluid losses from the body would lead to fatal dehydration within hours.

The filtration process of the kidney and the ultimate formation of urine is a complex process, but necessary to regulate blood volume and composition in order to maintain homeostasis. The main waste products excreted by the kidneys are urea, creatinine and uric acid. Urea is the main waste product and is produced during the breakdown of amino acids, whereas creatinine is produced by skeletal muscle during the breakdown of creatine phosphate, which plays an important role in muscle contraction. The more muscle bulk a person has, the higher their levels of creatinine will be. Typically, people of Afro-Caribbean descent will have higher levels of creatinine, as they have a higher muscle mass. This is important and should be taken into consideration when assessing the person's renal function and particularly when comparing the creatinine levels of an Afro-Caribbean person compared to a white Caucasian person. Uric acid is also produced daily as part of the recycling process of ribonucleic acid molecules (Martini and Karleskint 1998).

Diabetic nephropathy

Normal kidney function requires a very careful balance of reabsorption and secretion via a finely tuned filtration system. Disruption in kidney function has immediate effects on the constitution of the circulating blood and if the function of both kidneys becomes disrupted, death will occur within a few days if medical assistance is not provided.

Nephropathy as a complication of diabetes is characterized by the presence of albuminuria, hypertension and progressive renal insufficiency, ultimately leading to end-stage renal disease necessitating either renal dialysis or renal transplantation. Unfortunately, due to the close link between diabetic nephropathy and cardiovascular disease, many patients with type 2 diabetes who develop nephropathy will not reach the state of end-stage renal disease, as they will die of an acute cardiovascular episode first.

It is estimated that up to one-third of people with diabetes will die within the first year of dialysis and even those who are lucky enough to receive a renal transplant continue to have a higher mortality rate when compared to people who do not have diabetes. It has also been observed that the risk and mortality associated with cardiovascular disease increases as the nephropathy progresses (Fraser and Phillips 2007). The association between nephropathy, type 2 diabetes and cardiovascular disease is discussed later in the chapter.

Stages of nephropathy

1. Microalbuminuria
Diabetic nephropathy is clinically defined by the presence of proteinuria >500 mg/24 hours. This state is also referred to as overt nephropathy, proteinuria or macroalbuminuria, but it is now known that this is preceded by a state of microalbuminuria or incipient nephropathy.

The normal albumin excretion is 30 mg/24 hours, which is not detected on urine Albustix®, whereas microalbuminuria is diagnosed when the albumin excretion rate exceeds 30 mg/hour, but is less than 300 mg/hour. These levels are still not detectable on urine Albustix®. It is only when the albumin excretion exceeds 300 mg/hour that it can be observed on the Albustix®.

Key point

It is worth noting here that microalbuminuria refers to the amount of albumin that is excreted by the kidney and not that the albumin particles are smaller, as the term may suggest.

It is now widely accepted that the presence of microalbuminuria is the best predictive marker for the development of proteinuria and diabetic nephropathy, therefore it is no longer acceptable for the urine of people with diabetes to just be tested routinely with Albustix®, as these are clearly not sensitive enough. Microalbuminuria can now be detected using specific microalbumin urine dipsticks. These are more expensive than the routine Albustix®, but the benefits of identifying people with microalbuminuria will outweigh the costs if proteinuria can be prevented or delayed. Indeed, it is accepted that not all people with microalbuminuria will progress to proteinuria and nephropathy; some people will regress to normoalbuminuria if effective treatment can be instigated early in the disease process. This can only be achieved if appropriate screening that detects microalbuminuria is undertaken on an annual basis.

Alternative methods of identifying microalbuminuria and proteinuria are via a timed urine collection, but this is less convenient, requires a high level of patient compliance and as a result is prone to errors.

A positive urine test result for microalbuminuria should be repeated once or twice in the next month before a firm diagnosis is made. False-positive results can occur after heavy exercise or a urinary tract infection. Also, if a person develops heavy proteinuria over a short space of time then a reason other than diabetic nephropathy should be sought to explain this. Additionally, quick-onset proteinuria in the absence of retinopathy should be viewed with scepticism. This is because the cells in the blood vessels supplying the retina are the same size as the cells in the renal glomerulus. When damage to cells occurs, it will affect all the specific cells and will not be limited to the cells in just one location in the body.

2. Proteinuria

The link between proteinuria and diabetes has been known since the late 18th century and was further defined by Kimmelsteil and Wilson (1936, cited in Cooper 1998) in the 1930s, when a clear connection between proteinuria and hypertension was made. Twenty years later, physicians were beginning to realize that nephropathy was not a rare complication of diabetes, but actually affected up to 50% of people with diabetes.

More recently, it is estimated that about one-third of patients with type 1 diabetes will begin to develop the signs of kidney disease approximately 20 years after being diagnosed with diabetes (Schwarze and Dunger 2005).

The development of proteinuria has been shown to correlate specifically with an increase in the mesangium in the glomerulus. The mesangium is an inner layer of the glomerulus, which connects with the basement membrane surrounding the glomerular capillaries. The role of the mesangium is to support and anchor the capillary loops to enable them to retain their structure and function. It is made up of mesangial cells, which are phagocytic and often contain macromolecules or inflammatory agents which, when examined in a laboratory, aid in the diagnosis of kidney disease (Mosby's 2002).

It is thought that expansion of the mesangium reduces the capillary surface area available for filtration and therefore contributes to the progressive loss of renal function (Wolf *et al.* 2005). However, Wolf *et al.* (2005) are not convinced that expansion of the mesangium is the sole cause of the development of proteinuria in people with diabetes. They believe that changes also occur within the visceral layer of the Bowman's capsule, which give rise to alterations in the glomerular filtration barrier.

The parietal layer of the Bowman's capsule is constructed of simple squamous epithelium, which contributes to the structure of the capsule but has no role in the formation of filtrate. The visceral layer, on the other hand, clings and envelopes the glomerulus and is made up of specialist, highly modified branching epithelial cells called podocytes (Figure 7.3).

These cells resemble the shape of an octopus and terminate in foot processes that intertwine with one another as they adhere to the basement membrane of the Bowman's capsule (Marieb 2001). The foot processes of adjacent podocytes interdigitate and are separated by narrow spaces, which are bridged by a porous membrane called the slit diaphragm. These membranes contain pores that are highly permeable to water and small solutes, but generally impermeable to plasma proteins. The presence of proteinuria in people with diabetic nephropathy therefore suggests a dysfunction of the foot processes and slit diaphragm.

Further studies have shown that in patients with type 1 diabetes there is an increase in the width of the foot processes and in patients with both type 1 and type 2 diabetes the number and density of podocytes has been shown to be significantly reduced (Wolf *et al.* 2005). These findings have been further confirmed by the presence of podocytes in the urine of 80% of people with type 2 diabetes and proteinuria, while healthy control subjects had undetectable levels of urinary podocytes (Nakamura *et al.* 2000).

Podocytes have a limited capacity to replicate, so when they are lost they cannot be replaced with new cells. In order to compensate for this loss, the foot processes widen, reducing their ability to remain attached to the glomerulus basement membrane. This consequently creates 'bare' areas in the basement membrane, which results in proteinuria (Fioretto *et al.* 2007).

Other morphological changes are thought to occur in the podocyte. Smithies (2003) postulates that as the foot processes widen the slit diaphragm becomes

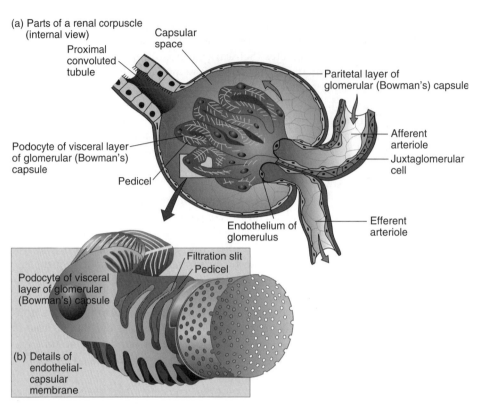

Figure 7.3 Formation of the Bowman's capsule and podocytes.

shorter, which may be a factor responsible for impeding the amount of water filtration and lowering the overall GFR, another sign of kidney damage.

Diabetic nephropathy and cardiovascular disease

Diabetic nephropathy has been categorized into different stages according to the values of urinary albumin excretion. Table 7.1 depicts the cut-off values adopted by the American Diabetes Association (2004, cited in Gross *et al.* 2005) for the diagnosis of micro- and macroalbuminuria and includes the main clinical features of each stage.

The close association between diabetic nephropathy and cardiovascular disease is clearly indicated in the table opposite, but the explanations offered for this are rather sketchy and appear to be poorly understood. One hypothesis is that people with diabetes who have just a slightly increased urinary albumin excretion rate may also have generalized vascular endothelium dysfunction.

As highlighted in Chapter 6, the endothelial layer of the body's vasculature has a vital role to play in the regulation of vessel tone and permeability, fibrinolysis

Table 7.1 Stage of diabetic nephropathy; cut-off values of urine albumin for diagnosis and main clinical characteristics (Gross *et al.* 2005).

Stages	Albumin cut-off values	Clinical characteristics
Microalbuminuria	20–199 µg/min	Abnormal nocturnal decrease of blood pressure and increased blood pressure levels
	30–299 mg/24 hours	Increased triglycerides, total and LDL cholesterol and saturated fatty acids
	30–299 mg/g*	Increased frequency of metabolic syndrome components
		Endothelial dysfunction
		Association with diabetic retinopathy, amputation, and cardiovascular disease
		Increased cardiovascular mortality
		Stable GFR
Macroalbuminuria	≥200 µg/min	Hypertension
	≥300 mg/24 hours	Increased triglycerides and total and LDL cholesterol
	>300 mg/g*	Asymptomatic myocardial ischaemia
		Progressive GFR decline

*Spot urine sample.
GFR, glomerular filtration rate; LDL, low-density lipoprotein.

and the synthesis of growth factors. Disturbance of these regulatory functions may not only cause atherothrombotic diseases but may also be associated with the development of proteinuria. Stehouwer *et al.* (1992) conducted a study to consider specifically whether there was a positive relationship between the presence of albuminuria, incidence of cardiovascular disease and endothelial dysfunction in people with type 2 diabetes. They concluded that a raised urinary albumin excretion level was only associated with an increased risk of new cardiovascular events when endothelial dysfunction was also present. It therefore appears that it is the endothelial dysfunction that is the main contributor to the development of microalbuminuria and subsequent cardiovascular complications.

Hypertension

Raised blood pressure is one of the key characteristics of diabetic nephropathy and eventually occurs in 85–90% of patients with chronic renal failure (Rennke and Denker 2007). In the early development of nephropathy, progression of the disease is rather slow, indicated by an initial GFR decline of 1.2 ml/minute/year. However, in the presence of hypertension that is not adequately treated, the rate of glomerular filtration decline is significantly accelerated to approximately

12 ml/minute/year (Greenstein *et al.* 2007), thus highlighting the importance of adequate blood pressure control in these people.

According to Cooper (1998), studies have shown that in animals with diabetes there is a measurable increase in the intraglomerular pressure, even in the absence of systemic hypertension. The renin–angiotensin system is thought to be responsible for this localized increase in pressure, as it has an important role to play in the regulation of blood pressure, urinary sodium excretion and renal haemodynamics.

Renin is an enzyme that is secreted by specialist cells in the afferent arteriole of each glomerulus. It is released in response to a decline in filtration rates, which may be due to a reduction in blood pressure, and acts by converting angiotensinogen, an α-globulin produced by the liver, into angiotensin I. Circulating angiotensin I is subsequently converted to angiotensin II by angiotensin-converting enzyme (ACE) in the capillary endothelial cells within the lungs. As angiotensin II is a powerful peripheral vasoconstrictor, it aims to increase renal perfusion by increasing blood pressure to maintain and improve a falling GFR. It also increases the release of antidiuretic hormone to create an increase in the amount of water reabsorbed in the distal convoluted tubules and collecting ducts of the kidney, again in an attempt to increase blood pressure. Antidiuretic hormone also works as a 'thirst transmitter' in the hypothalamus of the brain, encouraging the person to drink more to increase his or her intake of water and thus positively increase blood pressure levels.

In addition, angiotensin I is the principal hormonal stimulus for the production of aldosterone by the adrenal glands. Aldosterone increases the amount of sodium that is reabsorbed from the distal convoluted tubule and collecting ducts in exchange for an increased potassium excretion. The increase in sodium reabsorption leads to additional reabsorption of water by the kidney, which further increases blood pressure levels. Finally, as a protective mechanism to prevent blood pressure from being driven dangerously high, angiotensin II slowly reduces the amount of renin that is secreted.

It is also now known that angiotensin II can be synthesized at a variety of sites including the kidney, vascular endothelium, adrenal glands and the brain. It is therefore considered that within the kidney, locally generated angiotensin II is responsible for the rise in intraglomerular pressure without it affecting the renin–angiotensin system, as this would create a comparable rise in systemic blood pressure.

Case study: Winston

Winston is a 59-year-old black man of Afro-Caribbean origin. He has had type 2 diabetes for 17 years and has shown signs of diabetic nephropathy during the past 5 years. He is married to Takola and has two boys in their early 20s, who are currently fit and well.

He worked as a garage mechanic for a large motor company, but has had to take early retirement recently due to his diabetes and subsequent kidney disease. He has now developed end-stage renal failure and requires haemodialysis three times per week, which he has as an out-patient in a satellite dialysis unit. Having to give up work early has put quite a financial strain on the family and Winston feels to blame.

Past medical history

- Diagnosed with type 2 diabetes fifteen years ago but thinks that he probably had it at least a further five years prior to diagnosis.
- Diabetic retinopathy diagnosed 10 years ago and treated with pan-retinal laser therapy.
- Hypertension.
- Dyslipidaemia.
- No personal history of any cardiovascular events or stroke.
- Admits to smoking 20–30 low tar cigarettes per day.
- Obese, with a waist circumference of 109 cm and a body mass index (BMI) of 35.2 kg/m^2
- Regularly has an abnormally high haemoglobin A1c (HbA1c) level ranging between 10 and 12% but he does not undertake any blood glucose monitoring at home.

Family history

- Mother died aged 72 years from a debilitating cerebrovascular accident. She also had type 2 diabetes from the age of 50 years. This was generally poorly controlled and she regularly had HbA1c levels between 10 and 13.5%. She also had hypertension for which she was prescribed a range of different antihypertensive drugs but to no avail. Her compliance in taking numerous antidiabetes and antihypertensive agents was often questioned by healthcare professionals.
- Father had type 2 diabetes diagnosed when he was 44 years old. Five years after his initial diagnosis of type 2 diabetes he developed diabetic retinopathy and nephropathy and died at the age of 52 years of a fatal myocardial infarction (MI). Prior to his death his blood glucose control was poor and he often had an HbA1c result between 14 and 15%. He also required treatment for hypertension but was never able to achieve the required blood pressure targets. He had smoked cigarettes since being a teenager and was thought to smoke between 15 and 20 cigarettes per day. He never smoked cigars or pipe tobacco.
- Winston's father also required regular haemodialysis, for the treatment of end-stage renal disease due to his diabetes.

Continued

Medication

- Mixtard® 30, 64 units with his breakfast, 90 units with his evening meal.
- Metformin 850 mg three times a day with each main meal.
- Ramipril 5 mg once daily.
- Losartan 100 mg once daily.
- Nephro-Vite® one tablet daily.
- Aranesp® 4500 ng once a week, given intravenously.
- Venofer® 100 mg/dialysis session.
- Atorvastatin 40 mg once daily

Allergies

- None known.

Examination

- Blood pressure   150/90 mmHg.
- Pulse   80 bpm, regular.
- Temperature   37.0°C.
- Respirations   16/minute.
- Random capillary blood glucose level   15.1 mmol/l.
- HbA1c   11.4%.
- Total cholesterol   6.1 mmol/l.
- High-density lipoprotein (HDL)   0.8 mmol/l.
- Low-density lipoprotein (LDL)   3.5 mmol/l.
- Triglycerides   4.6 mmol/l.
- No longer passing urine.

Renal function blood tests – predialysis

- Sodium   138 mEq/l.
- Potassium   6.0 mEq/l.
- Creatinine   984 mg/dl.
- Urea   21 mg/dl.
- Chloride   97 mEq/l.
- Bicarbonate   25 mEq/l.
- Phosphate   1.62 mmol/l.
- Haemoglobin   12.6 g/dl.
- Ferritin   500 µg/l.

Discussion of Winston's case

The above case study depicting the healthcare scenario of Winston serves to illuminate a number of important predisposing factors relating to diabetic nephropathy. End-stage renal disease is particularly common in Afro-Caribbean people and it has been reported that they have a 4–25-fold greater risk of developing the disease than their white, Caucasian counterparts, which implies the presence of genetic and/or environmental risk factors (Bleyer *et al.* 2008). However, to date, no single gene has been clearly shown to be responsible for the increased susceptibility (Fraser and Phillips 2007).

Winston has a strong family history of type 2 diabetes with both his parents having the condition and he also has a family history of diabetic nephropathy, which his father developed. This is noteworthy as siblings from parents with diabetes with end-stage renal disease who subsequently also go on to develop diabetes are at an increased risk of developing end-stage renal disease themselves, as can be seen in Winston's history. In a study by Bleyer *et al.* (2008), a significant 46% of siblings with diabetes had microalbuminuria or macroalbuminuria. They also found that in a group of people who had been diagnosed with type 2 diabetes for between 0 and 5 years, 29% had at least microalbuminuria and 5.5% had overt proteinuria. In contrast, the UK Prospective Study showed a prevalence of microalbuminuria of 2.0% per year and 25% of people with type 2 diabetes developed microalbuminuria 10 years after being diagnosed with diabetes. In addition, macroalbuminuria occurs in 15–40% of patients with type 1 diabetes, with a peak incidence of around 15–20 years after diagnosis (Hovind *et al.* 2004). The findings in Bleyer *et al.*'s (2008) study therefore suggest that the duration of the person's diabetes may have been underestimated; none the less, end-stage renal disease remains a significant problem for patients with diabetes and their healthcare practitioners.

Further findings from Bleyer *et al.*'s (2008) study show that despite having family members receiving dialysis therapy, this does not seem to be a motivator for the sibling to minimize the risk factors for developing nephropathy, as 39.6% of the study participants were obese, 64.7% had hypertension and 57.4% had poor blood glucose control. Lack of access to healthcare could not be blamed for this, as over 80% of the siblings with diabetes saw a physician at least three times per year and 89.3% had medical insurance.

There now appears to be a consensus amongst healthcare professionals that patients who have developed persistent proteinuria will undoubtedly progress to end-stage renal failure, presuming that they survive the added cardiovascular risk burden associated with diabetic nephropathy (Fraser and Phillips 2007). Therefore, while genetic factors in the development of end-stage renal disease cannot be overlooked, inadequate blood glucose control and poor blood pressure control are also significant risk factors.

Blood glucose control

In both type 1 and type 2 diabetes, studies have shown that hyperglycaemia is a major determinant in the progression of diabetic nephropathy. Two large, landmark studies in diabetes, the Diabetes Control and Complications Trial (DCCT) (Diabetes Control and Complications Research Group 1995) and the UK PDS (Stratton *et al.* 2000) both showed that intensive glycaemic control could slow the development of diabetic nephropathy. Although both studies were conducted some time ago, the findings from them are still highly relevant within the field of diabetes care and management today.

The DCCT was a 10-year study involving 1441 people with type 1 diabetes throughout the USA and Canada. It was set up to compare the effects of an intensified insulin regimen versus a conventional, one or two insulin injections per day regimen, on the development and progression of diabetes-related complications. The results that emerged were so conclusive that the study was halted 1 year early.

The study randomly allocated people to either the 'intensive insulin treatment group' or the 'conventional insulin treatment group'. Those in the intensive insulin treatment group were set blood glucose targets of 3.9–6.7 mmol/l before meals and up to 10 mmol/l after meals. They were also given HbA1c targets of around 6% and were to achieve this via three or more doses of insulin per day and regular, four times per day blood glucose monitoring.

Conversely, those in the conventional insulin treatment group were to continue with their usual one or two insulin injections per day and monitor their blood glucose levels or urine for glycosuria once daily. The results showed that the intensive insulin treatment group had a massive 76% reduction in the risk of developing retinopathy, and the development of kidney disease was slowed among those who had early signs of the complication at the start of the study and then received intensive insulin treatment (Diabetes Control and Complications Research Group 1995).

The UKPDS is the largest clinical trial of type 2 diabetes ever conducted and provides conclusive evidence that the life-threatening complications of type 2 diabetes can be significantly reduced by appropriate treatment. The UKPDS was a 20-year study involving more than 5000 people with type 2 diabetes. Blood glucose and blood pressure levels were measured every 3 months in people across 23 centres throughout the UK. If blood pressure or blood glucose levels became raised above the agreed targets, current antihypertensive treatment doses were adjusted or new treatments were added.

The study clearly showed that people with type 2 diabetes are at an increased risk of developing complications if their HbA1c levels were regularly above 7.5%, or their blood pressure was greater than 150/85 mmHg. The figures in the study were broken down further to conclude that for every 1% reduction in HbA1c there was an associated 37% decrease in risk for microvascular complications and a 21% decrease in the risk of any end point or death related to diabetes (Stratton *et al.* 2000). These are significant results that cannot be ignored by healthcare practitioners working within diabetes care.

It is therefore no surprise that Winston has developed diabetic nephropathy as he has a strong individual and family history of poor blood glucose control, probably occurring over a long period of time. Indeed, there is no evidence to suggest that Winston has ever achieved optimal blood glucose control since being diagnosed as having diabetes.

While it may now seem to be too late for Winston to achieve optimal blood glucose control, the fact is that he is still a relatively young man at huge risk of cardiovascular disease, thus any achievement in blood glucose control must be beneficial. It would be recommended that he commence a basal/bolus insulin regimen, which would enable him to have greater control over his blood glucose levels, particularly as he now has to attend hospital for dialysis and his lifestyle is far from regular on a day-to-day basis.

As mentioned in Chapter 2, people who are taking a mixed insulin twice a day need to have predictable eating habits and lifestyle if blood glucose control is going to be achieved on this regimen. This will include having the same type and amount of food each day, eating at the same time of day and having the same amount of activity/exercise each day. Even though Winston is no longer working, his eating habits and lifestyle will differ between the days he receives dialysis and days when he does not, making his insulin requirements less predictable. A basal/bolus insulin regimen would give him the flexibility and freedom to alter his eating and lifestyle patterns accordingly and achieve better blood glucose levels on a regular basis.

Furthermore, a potential problem of taking a mixed insulin is that there is a danger of the person becoming hypoglycaemic mid-morning and just prior to lunch time (see Chapter 2). A mid-morning snack may be given on the dialysis unit, but lunch is generally not provided unless the person is attending another hospital department for an appointment the same afternoon. If the dialysis takes longer than expected, or hospital transport home is delayed, Winston is currently at risk of hypoglycaemia if he does not have his lunch at the usual time. By switching to a basal/bolus regimen, this would allow for greater flexibility in his eating times and thus reduce the risk of low blood glucose levels.

In being prescribed a basal/bolus regimen, Winston would be advised to take the long-acting, peakless insulin at his bedtime each night, as this time of day tends to be more regular for people. He would then inject the rapid-acting insulin each time he was about to eat either a main meal or a snack containing more than 10 g of carbohydrate.

On the mornings he attends the hospital for dialysis, if he has breakfast beforehand he will inject rapid-acting insulin with this and do the same if he has a mid-morning snack while on dialysis. The number of units of insulin injected would differ depending on the amount and type of carbohydrate eaten. It would be acceptable for Winston to then delay his lunchtime and only inject his insulin when his next meal is prepared and ready to eat. This would help alleviate potential stress and worry about having to eat at the same time each day and diabetes control would be enhanced as a result.

Oral sulphonylureas such as chlorpropamide or glibenclamide need to be prescribed and used with caution in people with diabetic kidney disease. As these drugs are predominantly excreted by the kidney, there is the potential that they can accumulate in renal failure, leading to prolonged and severe hypoglycaemia that can be potentially debilitating or fatal. Caution is also required when using thiazolidinediones in moderate or severe renal failure as they have a tendency to cause weight gain, which is a complication of renal failure and can lead to pulmonary oedema, cardiac failure and death.

With regards to his other medication, Winston is advised to take it as normal, first thing in the morning prior to his dialysis as most medications, including the ones Winston is prescribed, are not removed from the body system during the dialysis process.

Blood glucose monitoring

Winston will need to be taught the importance of regular self blood glucose monitoring and the appropriate actions to be taken if an abnormal reading, either high or low, is obtained. He will also need to be provided with the equipment to enable him to carry out this function. In giving patients choice, Winston should be shown a range of different blood glucose monitors and the relative merits and demerits of each clearly explained. An appropriate monitor should be selected that Winston finds easy and convenient to use. Taking the time to ensure that the monitor and its functions meet the needs of the individual patient will help to aid compliance in carrying out the required blood glucose monitoring.

Winston will be advised to monitor his blood glucose levels first thing in the morning before he has eaten anything (preprandially) to enable a fasting and baseline blood glucose level to be recorded. He will then need to conduct further blood glucose tests 2 hours after each of his main meals (postprandially). Studies have shown that the greatest benefit in reducing HbA1c levels can be achieved if blood glucose levels are consistently within the normal range of 4–7 mmol/l 2 hours postprandial (Woerle *et al.* 2006). He will need to record the blood glucose readings so that patterns and trends in blood glucose levels can be observed for, and treated if necessary, by either Winston or his healthcare team.

On the days Winston has dialysis, it would be prudent to record his blood glucose level as a predialysis assessment check to ensure that it is within target range. As the process of haemodialysis does not remove glucose from the blood and modern dialysate solution contains glucose, it is expected that Winston's blood glucose levels will remain stable throughout the procedure. Unless he becomes unwell, it is not necessary specifically to record his blood glucose levels again post-dialysis.

Hospital in-patients with diabetes on a renal ward will obviously need to have their blood glucose levels recorded more frequently, as they will be clinically unwell. In these circumstances, blood glucose levels should be recorded as advised for Winston when he is at home, preprandially first thing is a morning, and 2 hours postprandial. In addition, they would also need to be recorded at other times if the person became acutely unwell.

Patients treating their kidney disease with peritoneal dialysis may find that the accuracy of their home blood glucose testing is compromised. This is because some testing strips are subject to interference from maltose, icodextrin, galactose or xylase, which are found in some peritoneal dialysis fluids. In addition, the accuracy of some blood glucose meters is affected by changes in haematocrit, which is seen in renal failure. Inaccuracy of home blood glucose testing results should be suspected if they do not correlate with the person's HbA1c or with the random/fasting blood glucose samples tested by the laboratory.

Anaemia

In evaluating the effects of blood glucose control on long-term HbA1c levels, the complication of anaemia, which is a known problem in chronic kidney disease, needs to be considered. Anaemia is more severe in those with diabetes-related kidney disease and tends to develop earlier in the disease process (Conway *et al.* 2008). A strong correlation between anaemia and cardiovascular disease has also been reported but the precise mechanism of how anaemia may increase the risk of mortality in overt nephropathy has yet to be determined (Conway *et al.* 2008). However, Levin *et al.* (1999) report a linear relationship between the level of haemoglobin and left ventricular thickness. They found that, for each 0.5 g decrease in haemoglobin level, there was a 32% increase in left ventricular growth, thus significantly increasing the risk of the person experiencing an acute myocardial infarction (MI).

Erythropoietin is produced in the kidney in response to decreased oxygen delivery and is responsible for the production of mature red blood cells. The presence of anaemia normally induces a compensatory increase in erythropoietin production, but in renal failure this response is blunted due to the reduction of functioning renal tissue.

As there are less circulating red blood cells in a person with anaemia, glucose attached to the available red blood cells will be more concentrated. This makes it difficult to calculate accurately the actual/amended percentage of glucose attached to the haem part of the red blood cell, thus rendering the HbA1c blood results less reliable, with higher readings than normal. However, it is important to recognize that during the process of haemodialysis, red blood cells are not altered, 'washed' or removed, therefore dialysis *per se* will not affect the overall the person's overall HbA1c readings.

In recognizing the complication of anaemia, Winston is currently prescribed Aranesp® and Venofer® to boost his haemoglobin and ferritin levels.

Blood pressure control

The majority of people with type 2 diabetes have hypertension, which is strongly associated with the development and acceleration of diabetic nephropathy and also creates a greater increase in the risk of cardiovascular disease. However, the progression to diabetic nephropathy and the progression of microalbuminuria to macroalbuminuria can be delayed but interventions must be instituted early in the course of the disease process to be fully beneficial. This requires appropriate and timely screening and effective antihypertensive treatment as mentioned previously.

The BENEDICT study questioned whether the development of microalbuminuria could be reduced or even prevented (Vora and Weston 2006). In this study, 1209 patients were recruited to the double-blind study, and were randomized to one of four treatment regimens and followed-up for a median of 3.6 years. The researchers concluded that angiotensin-converting enzyme inhibitor (ACEI) therapy with trandolapril alone, or in combination with verapamil, can prevent the onset of microalbuminuria in patients with type 2 diabetes who are hypertensive but have a normal urinary albumin excretion. They went on to recommend that ACEIs could be a useful therapy in preventing the development of microalbuminuria and thereby reducing the risk of cardiovascular mortality and end-stage renal failure.

In the general management of type 2 diabetes, the National Institute for Health and Clinical Excellence (NICE) recommends that a person's blood pressure should be recorded at least annually in a person without previously diagnosed hypertension or renal disease (NICE 2008). If the blood pressure is at, or above, 140/80 mmHg it should be repeated at least twice within a 2 month period. Persistently raised blood pressure at, or above, 140/80 mmHg (or above 130/80 mmHg if there is kidney, eye or cerebrovascular damage) requires lifestyle and pharmacological management to reduce the levels and therefore the risk of kidney and cardiovascular disease.

The lowering of blood pressure on its own does have some benefits in delaying the progression of renal disease, but the key interventions for curbing progression of the disease also include reducing the level of albuminuria and blocking the renin–angiotensin system (RAS) (Mende 2006). Indeed, blocking the RAS has been shown to have beneficial effects on albuminuria, even in the absence of any reduction in blood pressure (Mogensen 2003).

Blood pressure goals of 130/80 mmHg are currently being recommended for all people with diabetes (American Diabetes Association 2004a, National Kidney Foundation 2004) but as lower blood pressures are associated with greater decreases in the level of proteinuria in people with renal disease, some renal consultants are recommending even lower blood pressure levels. Targets of 125/75 mmHg are being suggested for patients with very high levels of proteinuria, typically >1 g/dl (Mende 2006). Achieving these targets is not easy and patients often need to take a mélange of antihypertensive agents to achieve reductions in blood pressure.

Most antihypertensive agents currently on the market will generally reduce blood pressure to a similar extent, but they do not all exert the same effect on reducing albuminuria and protecting kidney function. Current hypertension guidelines (American Diabetes Association 2004b) recommend the use of ACEIs or angiotensin II receptor blockers (ARBs) as the preferred agents to use to help protect the kidney. Many have a preference for ACEIs in people with type 1 diabetes and ARBs in type 2 diabetes, although both have shown to reduce blood pressure and also block the RAS (Sawaki *et al.* 2008). This has the increased benefit of reducing proteinuria and delaying renal decline, but using only an ACEI or an ARB as monotherapy will often lead to incomplete RAS blockade.

Winston is taking ramipril, which is an ACEI, and losartan, an ARB. The theory underpinning this prescription is based on the information that ACEIs and ARBs block the RAS at different sites, therefore by using both types of drugs a more effective RAS blockade will be achieved (Kumar and Winocour 2005). Caution needs to be exercised in adopting this dual approach, with particular care given to monitoring the person's serum potassium (Fraser and Philips 2007).

Thiazide diuretics are also an option in treating hypertension, and NICE (2008) recommends them as a first-line treatment alongside calcium-channel blockers for high blood pressure in a persons of African-Caribbean descent. However, their use in patients with kidney disease is limited to those people who are still producing urine, hence Winston is not prescribed them.

Beta blockers such as atenolol are now used only as a fourth-line treatment intervention and with caution in renal disease. This is due to the reported side-effects such as dyslipidaemia, hyperglycaemia and weight gain when beta blockers are combined with a thiazide diuretic. They has also been associated with a slightly increased risk of death due to cardiovascular disease, stroke and MI (Kirby 2006); these risk factors are already present in those with type 2 diabetes and so need to be reduced rather than increased.

Other modifiable risk factors – smoking, lipids, dietary protein

In addition to reducing blood glucose levels and blood pressure to help delay the progression of diabetic nephropathy, there are other modifiable risk factors that Winston can adjust and control. He currently smokes 20–30 cigarettes per day, which some 25 years ago was demonstrated to be an independent variable for the development of microalbuminuria. Cigarettes exert their effects by increasing catecholamine levels, which worsen existing hypertension and microalbuminuria. Cigarette smoking has also been reported to be associated with a 2.2-fold increased risk for the progression of albuminuria, and overt proteinuria was found in 53% of smokers compared to 11% of non-smokers (Schwarze and Dunger 2005). Fraser and Philips (2007) comment that smoking accelerates progression at all stages of diabetic nephropathy and in addition is associated with a higher mortality rate for those on dialysis. It therefore goes without saying that smoking cessation advice and support should be commonplace to all healthcare professionals managing patients with diabetic nephropathy.

Low-protein diets have also been shown to reduce the progression of kidney disease in patients with diabetes. Toeller *et al.* for the EURODIAB IDDM Group (1997) recommend a protein intake of 20% of total energy or approximately 2 g/kg/day. Patients also need to follow a low-sodium, low-potassium, low-phosphate diet, which can be very restrictive for many people. In recognizing the amount of dietary restrictions imposed upon people, Winston would need to be seen by a dietitian and information should be given to him, and his wife, on the culture-specific foods he is able to eat freely, those he can eat in moderation and those foods he should ideally avoid.

In aiding compliance to a strict dietary regimen, it is a good idea not to restrict any foods completely, as this has the potential deleterious effect of making the person want them all the more. Therefore, it is more sensible to highlight the foods which, if eaten, should be done so only in very small quantities and not on a regular basis. In changing Winston's diet to comply with the recommendations, this may have a positive effect on his blood glucose levels. He would therefore need to be advised and encouraged to monitor his blood glucose levels more frequently during this transition period and continue to do so until his blood glucose levels became stable and within normal limits.

Fluids

In addition to a very restrictive diet, Winston will also be required to limit his fluid intake to approximately 1000 ml/day to prevent fluid overload and the development of pulmonary oedema. For some people this can be difficult to achieve but can be helped by the reduction of salt in the diet; however, this will not affect Winston's overall diabetes control or his day-to-day blood glucose levels.

Infection from fistula

Infection developing in the arteriovenous fistula is a potential concern for Winston. He is at an increased risk due to the need to puncture the skin a minimum of six times per week in order to site the cannulae for dialysis. A strict aseptic technique is therefore required and information on caring for the site and keeping it clean between dialysis sessions is needed. Regular observation of the puncture sites and fistula is also advised and any signs of infection reported immediately.

The presence of infection will have a direct effect on Winston's blood glucose levels causing them to rise, which will subsequently inhibit the healing process of the puncture sites in the fistula.

Diabetes monitoring and review

In managing the care of a person with diabetes who has developed end-stage renal disease, it is important to ensure that they still receive their routine diabetes screening and review. There is a tendency for people with diabetes who are being cared for by specialist teams to be neglected when it comes to having their 'routine' diabetes care needs addressed. This could mean that annual reviews and eye screening can be missed, resulting in retinopathy and diabetic eye disease not being diagnosed until it is too late to treat, with the potential devastating consequences of sight loss. In addition, foot disease may not be identified, which could lead to amputation that may have been avoided with prompt intervention and treatment.

Strategies therefore need to be in place to ensure that people with diabetes being cared for and managed by dialysis units still have access to, and are able to attend, their diabetes annual reviews. This may require the diabetes and renal teams putting into place alternative approaches for annual recall, review and screening for this client group.

Conclusion

This chapter has outlined the structure and physiology of the normal, healthy kidney and renal system and discussed how the presence of poorly controlled diabetes can lead to the devastating effects of end-stage renal disease as a result of developing diabetic nephropathy.

It has been shown that diabetic nephropathy is a serious, debilitating disease affecting a significant number of people with both type 1 and type 2 diabetes and the treatment and management of the condition accounts for a large proportion of healthcare costs. However, with the implementation of an effective screening programme in which the presence of microalbuminuria is tested for on an annual basis, and the prompt initiation of treatment, it is possible for some people to return to a state of normoalbuminuria and have the complications of renal disease halted.

The effects of blood pressure and blood glucose control on the incidence and development of renal disease have been studied in two large, diabetes landmark studies, the DCCT and the UKPDS. Each has shown a positive correlation between blood pressure and blood glucose control and the development and severity of diabetic nephropathy. Controlling these two factors and maintaining them within normal limits has been shown to have very positive benefits on the clinical outcomes of patients with diabetic nephropathy. Therefore, suggestions for controlling blood pressure and blood glucose have been offered and the need to self-monitor blood glucose levels on a regular basis emphasized.

The link between diabetic nephropathy and cardiovascular disease has also been explored and the significant consequences this can have for people with type 2 diabetes highlighted. In addition, the link between renal disease, anaemia and cardiovascular disease has also been discussed.

General management and discussion of a person with type 2 diabetes who has developed end-stage renal disease is given and includes issues relating to genetic factors, smoking, diet and lifestyle.

Diabetes and liver disease

Aims of the chapter

This chapter will:

1. Consider the link between diabetes and liver disease.
2. Discuss the pathophysiology of non-alcoholic fatty liver disease (NAFLD), its relationship to the metabolic syndrome and treatment.
3. Identify and discuss the aetiology of diabetes in patients with hereditary haemochromatosis.
4. Critically consider the care and clinical management of a person with liver disease and diabetes who is awaiting a liver transplant.
5. Describe and discuss the development and prevention of new-onset diabetes following organ transplantation.

When we consider diabetes and the mechanisms of blood glucose control, there is a tendency to just consider the pancreas and the balancing act provided by the alpha cells and the beta cells in the Islets of Langerhans to keep blood glucose levels within the normal range. However, in conjunction with skeletal muscle and adipose tissue, the liver is one of the principle organs involved in the metabolism of glucose and a link between diabetes and chronic liver disease was first noted in the first part of the 20th century.

The liver has a fundamental role in glucose homeostasis as it has the ability to convert glucose from the diet into glycogen and store it as a readily available energy supply. When energy is required, the liver will break down the stored glycogen via a process called glycogenolysis and release it into the blood stream via the portal vein. The liver is also able to manufacture 'new' glucose from an increased absorption of amino acids, thus increasing its function as an energy provider. This process is known as gluconeogenesis and also helps in maintaining glucose homeostasis. However, insulin is the key mediator in blood glucose control and any change in its secretion or action, results in the impairment of glucose metabolism. This can include enhanced glucose metabolism resulting in falling blood glucose levels, or impaired glucose metabolism where blood glucose levels will rise, causing complications if not treated promptly and effectively.

The association between chronic liver disease and impaired glucose metabolism has been well documented, with peripheral insulin resistance and altered pancreatic beta-cell function being identified as the primary mechanisms. Glucose metabolism is directly affected by conditions such as alcohol abuse, which leads to alcoholic hepatitis, liver steatosis found in non-alcoholic fatty liver disease (NAFLD), and portal hypertension, all of which cause reduced insulin clearance.

Alcohol-related liver disease

In recent years, moderate alcohol consumption, considered to be a maximum of 2–3 units per day for a woman and a maximum 3–4 units per day for a man (Department of Health 2006b), and in particular drinking red wine, has been shown to have a protective effect on insulin resistance and cardiovascular risk (van de Viel 2004); however, excessive alcohol intake is directly linked to impaired glucose metabolism. It is estimated that heavy drinkers have a two-fold increase in the risk of developing type 2 diabetes compared with moderate drinkers, as the toxic effect of chronic alcohol abuse causes pancreatic damage, resulting in impaired insulin secretion (Picardi *et al* 2006).

It has also been shown that even in the absence of pancreatic islet cell injury, long-term alcohol consumption markedly affects glucose control by directly impairing both lipid and carbohydrate metabolism (Picardi *et al*. 2006). Studies in alcohol-perfused rats have shown that ingestion of alcohol results in a decreased ability of the liver to convert glucose to glycogen (glycogenesis) and therefore to store glucose. It also causes increased glycogenolysis. These two faulty mechanisms serve to trigger and increase insulin resistance and ultimately cause a rise in blood glucose levels.

Liver damage due to excessive, chronic alcohol intake also causes a local, chronic inflammatory action where pro-inflammatory cytokines, such as tumour necrosis factor α (TNFα), interleukin-1β and interleukin-6, are released (Hoek and Pastorino 2002).

As in the inflammatory response found in cardiovascular disease, TNFα also plays a major role in the development of liver damage. Free fatty acids released from adipose tissue promote the synthesis of TNFα, which promotes hepatocellular death by altering levels of adenosine triphosphate (ATP) or increasing apoptosis. Secretion of TNFα also exacerbates insulin resistance as it causes an increased release of free fatty acids and TNFα from adipose tissue. Unsurprisingly, the level of TNFα secretion positively correlates with body mass index (BMI) – the higher the person's BMI, the more likely they are to have excess adipose tissue, with prime cells for the formation of TNFα (McAvoy *et al*. 2006).

Non-alcoholic fatty liver disease

As the levels of obesity rise in westernized society, so do the number of people who are diagnosed with type 2 diabetes. The link between NAFLD and diabetes is gradually becoming more widely known as the media report research, stories and case studies with increased frequency. However, what is not commonly acknowledged is the link between obesity, insulin resistance, type 2 diabetes and NAFLD. It is thought that between 80 and 90% of people who are obese and/or have type 2 diabetes will have NAFLD but in the majority of cases it does not progress to severe liver disease.

NAFLD is the term used to describe liver disease similar to that encountered in chronic alcohol abuse, but in the absence of alcohol. It encompasses a range of liver abnormalities from simple steatosis or fatty liver, non-alcoholic steato-hepatitis (NASH) and NAFLD-induced cirrhosis (McAvoy *et al.* 2006). In the majority of cases it is asymptomatic and only diagnosed by coincidence when a person has a liver function blood test.

The theory on the pathogenesis of NAFLD is still not fully understood but is based on the 'double-hit hypothesis' (Angulo 2002), which suggests a strong association with insulin resistance and features of the metabolic syndrome (see Chapter 6). In fact, NAFLD is considered to be a liver manifestation of the metabolic syndrome, with insulin resistance reported in all cases (McAvoy *et al.* 2006).

The first 'hit' is identified as the liberation of free fatty acids from peripheral tissues, as a result of insulin resistance and the counteractive increase in insulin secretion, which influxes into the liver. This in turn leads to excessive hepatic triglyceride production. Accumulation of the free fatty acids which cause oxidative stress characterizes the second 'hit'. This stimulates the release of TNFα, apoptosis and lipid peroxidation, causing cell damage.

NAFLD is particularly associated with central, rather than peripheral, obesity as visceral adipocytes are more prone to lipolysis. This is the process whereby lipids are broken down into their constituent fatty acids. The fatty acids produced are then released from central adipose sites and drain directly to the liver via the portal vein where they are 'fresh' and in abundance to cause damage to the liver. Damage includes the infiltration of fat cells into the hepatocytes, increasing the degree of hepatic insulin resistance and triggering a cyclical chain of events – as the liver disease advances, the degree of insulin resistance increases, and so on.

Non-alcoholic steatohepatitis

While NAFLD is considered to be a benign disorder, mainly diagnosed by an incidental pathological finding, it has been reported that NASH, a progression of NAFLD, can progress to advanced liver fibrosis in 20–30% of cases and may be related to numerous diagnoses of cirrhosis to which the cause is unknown or obscure. NASH may be asymptomatic for a long period of time and a significant number of people with the condition develop no specific symptoms. Although hepatomegaly is present in 75% of patients, a liver biopsy is the only way to distinguish NASH from the other liver disorders within the NAFLD spectrum (Yunianingtias and Volker 2006).

In the early stages of NAFLD, the liver cells become filled with multiple fat droplets. At this stage, the number and size of fat droplets in the liver cells is not sufficient to displace the centrally located cell nucleus. However, as the condition progresses and NASH develops, the size of the fat cells increases and they push the nucleus to the periphery of the cell wall, creating a classic 'signet-ring' appearance. During tissue processing, the fat cells dissolve leaving empty, well-delineated vesicles. It is the presence of these vesicles on biopsy that aids in the diagnosis of NASH.

According to Guidorizzi de Siqueira *et al.* (2005) approximately 50% of patients with NASH will develop liver fibrosis, 20% develop cirrhosis and 3% will progress to end-stage liver failure. Specific risk factors have been identified that help predict the development of progressive fibrosis, characterized by the formation of scar tissue in response to liver damage, which leads to cirrhosis in patients with NAFLD. Obesity and diabetes are considered to be the strongest predictors, but other factors include: (1) advancing age; (2) high alanine transaminase levels and also the ratio of aspartate aminotransferase to alanine transaminase more than 1; (3) hypertension; and (4) hypertriglyceridaemia (Angulo *et al.* 1999).

When the additional complication of type 2 diabetes is added to the equation, this has been found to accelerate the progression of fibrosis to cirrhosis in a person with NASH. Furthermore the presence of NASH in a person with type 2 diabetes has been shown to further increase the risk for cardiovascular disease in this already high-risk population (Hickman *et al.* 2008). A study by Targher *et al.* (2005), which considered the risk of a cardiovascular disease in patients with NAFLD and type 2 diabetes, found that the risk of cardiovascular events in this population was significantly increased, even when raised liver enzymes and the metabolic syndrome were not present. This increased risk needs to be appreciated by healthcare professionals and could act as an indicator to actively screen for NAFLD in people with type 2 diabetes, rather than leaving the diagnosis to chance. By doing this, preventative treatment can be instigated early in the disease process and the progression of the liver disease halted.

Treatment of non-alcoholic fatty liver disease

As NAFLD has very close links with the metabolic syndrome, it is not surprising that that the main treatment strategies will be congruent with the treatment options offered to those with type 2 diabetes and cardiovascular disease. There are four main strategies to be employed in the prevention and treatment of NAFLD, namely lifestyle intervention, treatment of dyslipidaemia, increasing insulin sensitivity and the use of antioxidant/anticytokine agents (McAvoy *et al.* 2006).

Lifestyle intervention

Lifestyle interventions aimed at reducing insulin resistance are of paramount importance in treating NAFLD. As the majority of patients are overweight or obese, they are strongly advised to follow a weight-reducing diet. While a reduction of just 10% body weight will have positive benefits on blood pressure, cholesterol, alanine transaminase levels and a reduction in the development of steatosis, patients need to be encouraged and motivated to continue weight loss until their BMI is within the 'normal' range (18.5–24.9 kg/m^2).

Waist circumference is now deemed more important than measurements of BMI as a waist measurement of >80 cm for women or >94 cm for men is an indicator of visceral fat causing peripheral insulin resistance. Ideally, patients need to lose sufficient weight to achieve a 'healthy' waist circumference, as this will impact significantly on reducing levels of insulin resistance and therefore increasing insulin sensitivity. However, the rate at which excess weight is shed in people with NAFLD needs to be considered. Yunianingtias and Volker (2006) report that rapid weight loss in this group could have the detrimental effect of exacerbating the degree of fibrosis and inflammation, therefore a weight loss of 0.5–1 kg per week is considered to be safe and effective.

Contrary to this, Dixon *et al.* (2004) found that patients with NAFLD who underwent bariatric surgery in the form of gastric banding for obesity did not experience portal or lobular inflammation, despite having a large and quite rapid weight loss. They went on to consider whether following a very low-calorie diet or having gastroplasty results in significant malabsorption leading to nutritional deficiencies and alterations in intestinal flora, which have been found to increase liver fibrosis.

Diets rich in saturated fat and unsaturated lipids and low in carbohydrates have been found to contribute to the rapid development of NASH, as the fat content is thought to increase oxidative stress and promote liver injury. Patients should therefore be advised to eat a 'healthy diet' in which a maximum of 35% of the total energy is derived from fat intake (Lieber *et al.* 2004). This will help to protect liver function and will facilitate gradual weight loss.

Unfortunately, lifestyle interventions are notoriously difficult to execute and maintain over long periods of time. Over recent years, the pharmaceutical industry has capitalized on this huge growth area and produced three different drugs, orlistat, sibutramine and rimonabant, which are now licensed in Europe for the treatment of obesity. When used as monotherapy they are able to yield weight loss results, but they have been shown to work more effectively when combined with lifestyle modification (Wadden *et al.* 2005). This goes to prove that taking anti-obesity medication only augments the actions of lifestyle changes and does not replace them. Drug therapy should not be considered as a license to eat large portions of food or high-fat, high-calorie foods.

Lifestyle changes should also include regular exercise. This is defined as 20–30 minutes of planned exercise on a minimum of 5 days per week (Evans *et al.* 2004). As mentioned in earlier chapters, walking of moderate intensity is an excellent mode of exercise, particularly for people with diabetes. Regular, brisk walking has been shown to reduce body fat, decrease insulin resistance and improve blood lipid control (Foreyt and Poston 1999). Unfortunately, the benefits of exercise are only short lived, which is why people are encouraged to build in some form of exercise on most days of the week to reap the most benefit.

While regular walking can be incorporated into a person's daily routine relatively simply, for the person with diabetes, specific medical issues and precautions need to be considered. Attention needs to be given to the increased risk of the person experiencing a hypoglycaemic episode during, or up to 15 hours after, exercise. This delay in hypoglycaemia is due to the liver and skeletal muscle needing to 'refuel', i.e. replenish glycogen stores to ensure a continuous supply of energy is readily available. Patients with diabetes who are taking a sulphonylurea or prescribed insulin therapy are most at risk if they do not take into account the effect of exercise on their blood glucose levels. As the action of sulphonylureas is to increase insulin production from the pancreatic beta cells, too much insulin may be produced to meet the body's needs if exercise has already reduced blood glucose levels. Similarly, the amount of subcutaneous insulin to be injected would also need to be reduced, in order to overt a hypoglycaemic episode. People therefore need to be clearly educated on the effect of their medication and exercise on controlling their own blood glucose levels and avoiding hypoglycaemia.

Treatment of dyslipidaemia

The role of statin therapy in NAFLD is unclear. Ordinarily, statin therapy would be contraindicated in a person with liver disease, as it can occasionally lead to muscle and liver toxicity. Generally, hepatotoxicity from statins tends to be mild but instances of marked liver injury have been reported in a few cases. For these reasons, manufacturers recommend that people without liver disease have a liver function test performed within 6 months of commencing statin therapy to rule out the presence of any abnormal liver function tests, which may be exacerbated by the therapy. They also recommend that statins are not prescribed to patients who have persistent elevated transaminase levels.

As NAFLD is strongly associated with insulin resistance and the metabolic syndrome, these people are at a hugely increased risk of having a fatal cardiovascular event. This risk can be significantly reduced by lowering lipid levels via diet and statin therapy. The benefits of statin therapy therefore need to be counterbalanced against the potential deterioration of the liver disease.

A study by Chalasani et al. (2004) specifically evaluated whether individuals with elevated baseline liver enzymes were at a higher risk of developing hepatotoxicity with statin use. Three cohorts, totalling 4024 patients, were used in the study, which found that the frequency of mild to moderate or severe elevations of liver enzymes in patients with already higher than normal liver enzymes, who were prescribed statin therapy, was not significantly higher that that of the patients with elevated liver enzymes, who were not prescribed a statin. Their data also showed that some individuals with high baseline liver enzymes also have elevations in their liver biochemistries, regardless of whether or not statins are prescribed. Chalasani *et al.* (2004) concluded that individuals with elevated liver enzymes do not have an increased susceptibility to hepatotoxicity from statins, giving confidence to practitioners to prescribe them in patients with liver disease and dyslipidaemia.

Increasing insulin sensitivity

As already mentioned, patients with NAFLD have a high propensity to peripheral insulin resistance, which contributes to the development of liver steatosis and fibrosis. It therefore seems appropriate to target this with the use of insulin sensitizing agents, such as metformin and/or thiazolidinediones. Studies have shown both these agents to be effective in increasing insulin sensitivity in patients with liver disease, resulting in reduced alanine transaminase levels and a decrease in liver volume.

In considering the use of metformin in NAFLD, Bugianesi *et al.* (2005) demonstrated that the use of metformin could increase the chances of returning alanine transaminase levels to within the normal range, and it has been shown to decrease body weight and BMI. It has also been linked to a decrease in liver volume and liver fat but, to achieve maximum benefits, it needs to be coupled with nutritional counselling.

Unfortunately, both these drugs have significant side-effects, including gastrointestinal disturbances with metformin and considerable weight gain and anaemia with the thiazolidinediones; these side-effects may be enough to affect compliance and continuation of treatment. If this is the case and treatment is stopped, it has been shown that alanine transaminase levels will rise again.

Antioxidant/anticytokine agents

Vitamin E, beta-carotene and petoxifylline, a TNFα inhibitor, are among the main agents in this class. While some positive benefits have been observed in the use of vitamin E and pentoxifylline to reduce alanine transaminase, there is currently no robust evidence to support these claims.

Other potential therapies

Angiotensin II, which is the main peptide of the renin–angiotensin system (RAS), regulates cell growth, inflammation and fibrosis, all of which are abnormally present in NAFLD, indicating that RAS has a role in liver disease. Hirose *et al.* (2007) studied the role of an angiotensin II type 1 receptor blocker (ARB) in rats with NASH. Their findings concluded that the use of an ARB dramatically suppressed liver fibrosis in these rats by up to 70%. This is a promising potential agent as a preventative therapy for NASH but further *in vivo* studies need to be conducted.

Links have also been made between the presence of bacterial overgrowth in the gut and an increase in cytokine concentrations in the portal vein, which increases hepatic inflammation. Antibiotics and probiotics have been used in attempts to alter bowel flora and in a rodent model, probiotics have successfully reduced TNFα concentrations and therefore hepatic inflammation (Li *et al.* 2003).

Hepatitis C

Co-existing liver damage from infections such as hepatitis C can lead to more progressive forms of NAFLD, in which hepatic fibrosis develops at a much faster and aggressive rate. With this comes the increased risk of developing hepatocellular carcinoma. In addition, it appears that people with hepatitis C are at a 70% higher risk of developing type 2 diabetes than those without hepatitis C infection, and the diabetes tends to develop at a younger age compared to age-group counterparts without hepatitis C (Wang *et al.* 2007). Indeed, Wang *et al.* (2007) found that the diabetogenic effect of hepatitis C infection was approximately equal to the effect of overweight and obesity as risk factors for type 2 diabetes. Antonelli *et al.* (2005) on the other hand, found that patients with hepatitis C infection and type 2 diabetes presented with a lower BMI than their counterparts with hepatitis C but not diabetes. Interestingly, hepatitis B has not been linked to the development of type 2 diabetes (Wang *et al.* 2007).

The mechanism by which hepatitis C infection causes type 2 diabetes is not fully understood yet, but it is hypothesized that the presence of the hepatitis virus causes defects in the insulin signalling pathways, which reduce the amount of insulin secreted. The hepatitis C virus has also been found in the pancreatic beta cells; this causes alterations in their function and ultimately defects in insulin secretion (Wang *et al.* 2007). These factors therefore contribute to rising blood glucose levels and the development of type 2 diabetes.

These findings have huge implications for public health worldwide. The prevalence of hepatitis C virus is endemic in some developing countries, potentially impacting on the already fast-rising numbers of people being diagnosed with type 2 diabetes across the globe. Actions taken to help reduce the risk of diabetes, such as weight loss and lifestyle modification, should also be emphasized to those with hepatitis C infection, to help prevent or delay the onset of type 2 diabetes. People with hepatitis C infection also need to be screened for type 2 diabetes on a regular basis and starting at an earlier age according to Wang *et al.*'s (2007) findings.

Hereditary haemochromatosis

Hereditary haemochromatosis (HH), sometimes termed genetic haemochromatosis, is a disease of the liver but is not associated with NAFLD or NASH. It is defined by the European Association for the Study of the Liver (EASL 2000a) as a condition in which iron accumulates in the liver, pancreas, heart and other organs, impairing their structure and function. It is a condition with widespread prevalence amongst the Caucasian population, in particular those of northern European descent.

The iron accumulation that occurs in HH is due to a genetic mutation of the HFE C282Y gene on chromosome 6. This is the most common homozygous mutation accounting for up to 90% of all cases in the UK (Tavill 2001) and was identified in 1996 by Feder *et al*. (1996). It affects three times more men than women, with premenopausal women being more protected due to regular blood loss via monthly menstruation and pregnancy.

Early symptoms of the condition include fatigue, arthralgia and abdominal pain; if left untreated, later classical symptoms develop including liver cirrhosis, diabetes mellitus, impotence and cardiac failure.

Diagnosis of HH is made via a number of specific blood tests pertaining to iron level. Serum ferritin is an indicator of the level of iron stored in the body, but in the early stages of HH these levels are not necessarily raised. They do not tend to exceed the upper limits of normal until storage of iron in the liver is excessive – once this is reached serum ferritin rises disproportionately with the degree of liver damage (Clayton and Holt 2006).

Transferrin saturation is a more sensitive and specific test for iron accumulation and is derived from the serum iron concentration and the total iron binding capacity, from which the percentage saturation is then calculated. An upper limit of 55% in men and 50% in women indicates iron accumulation (British Society for Haematology 2000).

Treatment is usually by phlebotomy using venesection, where 400–500 ml of blood is removed each week initially, equating to 200–250 mg of stored iron. This process is repeated until the serum ferritin has reduced to 20–50 µg/l and transferrin saturation is below 30% (EASL 2000b). Once these levels have been achieved, maintenance venesection will take place every few months to preserve these biochemical levels. As potentially large amounts of blood are being removed, it is important to also monitor haemoglobin levels to ensure that the patient does not become anaemic.

HH is now clearly linked to diabetes, but the underlying pathophysiology is not fully understood, although evidence suggests that the main causative factor is insulin deficiency due to poor functioning and a reduced number of pancreatic beta cells (McClain *et al*. 2006). As the mechanisms for developing diabetes secondary to HH are not related to those that typically produce type 1 and type 2 diabetes (see Chapter 1) the American Diabetes Association classifies this type of diabetes under the heading of 'other specific' (American Diabetes Association 2006). Owing to this non-standardized classification of the condition, routine management approaches for type 1 or type 2 diabetes may be difficult to apply, therefore treatment needs to be based around an individualized assessment of the patient.

Specifically, when discussing diet and the need to follow a 'healthy' eating plan with the person with diabetes and HH, account needs to be taken of the dietary recommendations from the Haemochromatosis Society (2006). These include the avoidance of iron-rich foods, tonics containing iron and fortified breakfast cereals. Patients should be encouraged to drink tea with a meal, as this reduces the amount of iron absorbed and does not affect blood glucose levels.

Regular exercise will also feature as part of the management of diabetes, but consideration needs to be given to any co-morbidities the patient may have, such as cardiac dysfunction or joint pain, which can be a complication of both diabetes and HH.

Additionally, patients with diabetes and HH are at increase risk of hypo-glycaemia if they are receiving insulin therapy or are prescribed a sulphonylurea, as both can result in an overdose of either exogenous or endogenous insulin. The glucose counter-regulation mechanism, which stimulates the liver to release stored glucose when blood glucose levels fall, may be impaired in these people due to the iron overload infiltrating pancreatic alpha cells and liver cells. This may lead to unpredictable and more severe hypoglycaemia, which the patient will need to be able to identify through self blood glucose monitoring.

The reliability of the haemoglobin A1c (HbA1c) as a blood test to monitor overall diabetes control will be reduced in these people. Regular venesection, which these people require, will remove red blood cells to which glucose has attached itself. It will therefore be difficult to estimate how much glucose has been removed during venesection and what percentage of glucose has become attached to the red blood cells over the previous 3-month period. In this instance a fruc-tosamine blood test may be recommended; this is able to give an indication of the person's blood glucose levels over the preceding 14–21 days. This test is suitable for people who have experienced blood loss, have had rapid changes in their dia-betes treatment or are pregnant and require very careful blood glucose monitoring to prevent the occurrence of fetal abnormalities.

As the fructosamine reference values are dependent on a number of different factors, a standard reference range is not available for this test. Patient's age, gender and test method have different meanings in different laboratories, therefore the specific reference range provided by the laboratory will be individualized to the patient.

Additionally, home blood glucose monitoring would be strongly advised in these circumstances, with the patient recording their blood glucose levels prepran-dially, first thing in the morning before they eat or drink, and 2 hours postpran-dial. Further monitoring would be advised if the patient felt unwell. The importance of accurately recording the results and bringing them to clinic for review would need to be emphasized so that they could be compared with the results of the fructosamine blood test.

Additionally, as the regular venesection will remove glucose from the blood, this will impact on the person's blood glucose levels. As a result they may need to reduce the amount of insulin they take or the dose of sulphonylurea, in order to avoid hypoglycaemia. Again, regular, self blood glucose testing in this instance will enable treatment to be titrated to body need.

Case study: Paul

Paul is a 50-year-old man who was diagnosed with type 2 diabetes 8 years ago but he suspects that he had the condition at least a further 2 years before being formally diagnosed. Four years ago, as a result of routine liver function tests, he was diagnosed as having NAFLD and approximately 1 year ago; this developed into NASH. He has portal hypertension and has abdominal ascites for which he requires paracentesis approximately every 4 weeks. This requires him to attend hospital for just an overnight stay if the paracentesis procedure is successful with no complications. He is on the waiting list for a liver transplant.

Past medical history

- Type 2 diabetes.
- Hypertension.
- Ascites, which is causing him to be short of breath.
- Portal hypertension.
- Not currently showing signs of encephalopathy.
- Has developed oesophageal varices, but has not experienced bleeding from these to date.
- Dyslipidaemia.
- Experienced an acute inferior myocardial infarction (MI) aged 48 years. This was causing him to experience slight shortness of breath on exertion prior to the development of the ascites.
- Does not smoke and has never smoked.
- Classed as overweight. Waist circumference and BMI are difficult to estimate owing to presence of ascites, but BMI is thought to be approximately 35.3 kg/m^2.
- Diabetes control could be improved as his HbA1c results taken every 6 months have ranged from 8.2 to 10.1% over the past 2 years. Paul does monitor his blood glucose levels at home, but is unsure how to counteract or avoid an abnormally high reading. He reports that his blood glucose levels are generally between 8 and 13 mmol/l when he takes them at different times of the day.

Family history

- Mother aged 80 years is still alive but living in a nursing home due to being in the advanced stages of senile dementia.
- Mother has been receiving treatment for hypertension for the past 20 years and as a result her blood pressure is well controlled.
- She does not have diabetes or signs of dyslipidaemia.

- Other than the senile dementia, she is generally fit and well and remains fully mobile.
- Father died aged 62 years with a fatal MI. He had experienced angina for 10 years prior to this. While he was not diagnosed as having type 2 diabetes, Paul always suspected that he may have had the condition, which may have contributed to his death.

Medication

- NovoMix®25, 50–60 units with breakfast, 85–90 units with evening meal.
- Metformin 850 mg three times a day with each main meal.
- Irbesartan 300 mg once daily.
- Pravastatin 40 mg once daily taken at night.
- Spironolactone 200 mg daily.
- Propranolol 80 mg twice daily.
- Isosorbide mononitrate 40 mg twice daily.

Allergies

- None known.

Examination

- Blood pressure   140/80 mmHg.
- Pulse   72 bpm, regular.
- Temperature   37.0°C.
- Respirations   22/minute.
- Random capillary blood glucose level 11.3 mmol/l.
- HbA1c   9.4%.
- Total cholesterol   5.2 mmol/l.
- High-density lipoprotein (HDL)   1.4 mmol/l.
- Low-density lipoprotein (LDL)   2.3 mmol/l.
- Triglycerides   4.8 mmol/l.

Liver function tests

- Total bilirubin   70 μmol/l.
- Alkaline phosphatase   350 units/l
- Albumin   28 g/l.
- Alanine transaminase   55 units/l.

Discussion of Paul's case

Management of Paul's liver disease while he is awaiting a suitable liver donor needs to focus on alleviating the ascites, reducing the portal hypertension and increasing his insulin sensitivity, therefore reducing his risk of cardiovascular disease.

1. Ascites

Ascites is the accumulation of fluid in the peritoneal cavity and is commonly associated with cirrhosis and severe liver disease. Patients with mild ascites may not be aware of the condition, but as the amount of fluid in the peritoneal cavity builds up, the abdomen becomes increasingly distended and patients will complain of a progressive abdominal heaviness and pressure. They will become increasingly short of breath as the increased pressure impinges on the diaphragm.

Ascites can be determined via physical examination of the abdomen, which will display bulging of the flanks. There will also be a difference in the note obtained when the flanks are percussed with the patient in a reclined position, compared to when they are turned on their side. Additionally, in severe ascites a 'fluid wave' can be felt. This is where pushing or tapping on one side of the abdomen will create a 'wave-like' effect through the fluid, which can then be felt on the opposite side of the abdomen. A diagnosis is confirmed via a diagnostic paracentesis in which the fluid is reviewed for its gross appearance, protein level, albumin and red and white blood cell count. An ultrasound scan can also be used to diagnose the presence of ascites.

Treatment is aimed at the symptoms which result from the presence of ascites and generally involves regular drainage of fluid from the peritoneal cavity. The accumulation of further fluid can be slowed by the patient following a no-added-salt diet. This treatment modality can be effective in up to 15% of patients.

Aldosterone is a hormone that acts to increase salt retention, therefore it seems sensible to instigate medication that counteracts the effects of the aldosterone. Thus, Paul has been prescribed spironolactone, which blocks the action of the aldosterone receptor in the collecting tubule of the kidney. If this is not sufficient, a loop diuretic such as frusemide can be added. Potassium levels and renal function should be monitored closely while the patient is on these medications.

2. Portal hypertension

The portal vein is formed by the union of the splenic vein and the superior mesenteric vein and divides into a left and right branch before it enters the liver. Unlike other veins, which drain blood from the body to the heart, the portal vein drains blood into the liver and not from the liver. Almost all of the blood from the digestive system drains into the portal vein and into the liver, where it is filtered and toxic substances are removed, before the blood enters the general circulatory system.

The portal vein divides and subdivides many times to form a number of smaller vessels, which open into hepatic sinusoids. Once the blood collected in the sinusoids has been through the liver's detoxification process, it is recollected into the hepatic vein and enters the inferior vena cava and ultimately the circulatory system.

Portal hypertension is a raised blood pressure in the portal vein and its branches. It occurs as a result of a resistance to the flow of blood through the portal system, which results in blood being forced down alternative channels. Resistance is caused by ascites and hepatic encephalopathy, among other things, and is often defined as a portal pressure gradient of 5 mmHg or more.

Paul has been prescribed propanolol and isosorbide mononitrate in attempts to reduce the level of hypertension, but this treatment regimen needs to be prescribed with caution as there is a risk of deterioration in liver function with the use of propanolol. Another treatment option is transjugular intrahepatic portosystemic shunting, in which a connection is made between the portal system and the venous system. The aim of this is based on the pressure in the venous system being lower than that in the portal system, thus decreasing the pressure over the portal system and a decreased risk of complications.

The presence of portal hypertension can result in reduced insulin clearance. This can have significant implications for Paul and the management of his type 2 diabetes and is compounded by the insulin resistance, which requires high levels of circulating insulin in order to have an effect on lowering blood glucose levels.

Endogenous insulin is normally broken down and removed from the circulation within approximately 15 minutes of being secreted, to prevent high levels of insulin building up in the blood and causing the person to become hypoglycaemic. The speed at which exogenous insulin is broken down will be dependent on the type of insulin that has been injected. Different insulins can remain in the blood stream for as little as 2 hours or for over 24 hours. Reduced insulin clearance as a result of portal hypertension could result in excess amounts of insulin remaining active, thus increasing Paul's susceptibility to serious hypoglycaemia.

Paul needs to be informed of the signs and symptoms of impending hypoglycaemia and know how to treat a low blood glucose level effectively. He also needs to ensure that he informs others of his condition by wearing a medic alert chain. Regular self blood glucose monitoring will be required on a daily basis, and at times during the night, to identify the action of the circulating insulin on blood glucose levels and to avert hypoglycaemia.

Blood glucose levels may also appear erratic due to the reduced insulin clearance. In these circumstances multiple daily injections via a basal/bolus insulin regimen or commencement on insulin pump therapy would provide Paul with an easier and more flexible way of treating his diabetes. Using a fast-acting insulin that is cleared from the blood stream quickly would help to limit the degree of insulin build-up, which could occur more readily with longer-acting insulin preparations. This type of insulin regimen, coupled with education on the action of insulin and the link between diet, exercise and blood glucose levels, would also help Paul to improve his overall glycaemic control and would lower his risk of developing diabetes-related complications, in particular his increased risk of cardiovascular disease.

In addition to a reduced insulin clearance, a person with advanced liver disease may also experience difficulties controlling their blood glucose levels, as the damage found in cirrhosis stops the liver from storing glycogen, which is needed for energy. In this case patients may be advised to eat small meals often. This will provide the body with a more continuous supply of energy, which will prevent it from breaking down muscle protein to provide energy between meals.

For the person with diabetes, this eating pattern will undoubtedly affect their blood glucose levels and diabetes control. Again a basal/bolus regimen or insulin pump therapy would be the most suitable treatment option for these people. Small amounts of insulin can be given with each snack/meal to control the rise in blood glucose level that the food will generate. This will have a positive effect on overall blood glucose control and will help to prevent hypo- or hyperglycaemia from occurring.

New-onset diabetes following transplantation

Liver transplantation has transformed the lives of many people with liver disease and Paul is certainly looking forward to the prospect of receiving a new liver and an increased quality of life. Organ transplantation requires immunosuppressive therapy to help prevent graft rejection, but the potent immunosuppressive agents currently used are host to a number of significant side-effects for the patient. These include nephrotoxicity, neurotoxicity, hypertension, weight gain, hyperglycaemia and in some cases, new-onset diabetes mellitus.

New-onset diabetes following liver transplantation (NODAT) was as high as 46% before the use of newer, more advanced immunosuppressive agents, such as cyclosporine A in the 1980s and tacrolimus in the 1990s. The previous high incidence was thought to be largely due to the use of high-dose steroid therapy to prevent organ rejection. The incidence of NODAT today is currently at about 15% (Marchetti 2005), which is a huge improvement but still means that a significant number of people are developing diabetes post-organ transplantation.

A careful and through assessment is an essential part of the transplant procedure, as the function of all of the body's organs and their ability to withstand the stress of a major operation and long anaesthesia time needs to be determined. Included in the assessment should be screening to identify those patients who are most at risk of developing NODAT post-transplant. High-risk groups have been identified; these include a strong family history of diabetes among first-degree relatives, being of non-white ethnicity (Bäckman 2004) and increasing age at the time of transplantation. Obesity is also included in the list of predisposing factors, as well as pre-existing hypertension. It has also been reported in the literature that individuals who have received a liver transplant due to hepatitis C have a 40% increased risk of developing diabetes post-transplant (Soule *et al.* 2005). This is thought to be due to an increase in insulin resistance caused by the hepatitis C virus resulting in pancreatic beta-cell dysfunction.

Additionally, in these instances the stress of living with a chronic illness, impending surgery and the prospect of a transplant should not be underestimated; this can play a major role in the development of type 2 diabetes as psychological stress further increases insulin resistance.

However, while these risk factors are acknowledged as potentially contributing to the development of diabetes in the post-transplant phase, it also needs to be recognized that the above factors are also high-priority risk factors for the development of type 2 diabetes, independent of liver disease and transplantation. Therefore, it needs to be questioned whether these patients would have gone on to develop diabetes anyway, regardless of whether or not they had received a liver transplant and commenced on immunosuppressant therapy.

The screening of patients preoperatively should include identifying those most at risk of developing NODAT and also those patients who may already have type 2 diabetes but not know it, as they are yet to develop symptoms and become diagnosed. This would enable appropriate diet, lifestyle and antidiabetes treatments to be commenced preoperatively to ensure that the patient is metabolically stable at the time of surgery. It would also help to reduce the risk of intra- and postoperative complications, such as hypo- and hyperglycaemia, infection and poor wound healing.

Cardiovascular disease has been shown to be the leading cause of death in post-transplant patients whose graft had been functioning well (Bäckman 2004). As Paul has a previous history of MI he will require specific attention and management to ensure that his cholesterol levels, blood pressure and blood glucose levels are kept within 'safe' parameters preoperatively and following surgery.

Those patients deemed to be at high risk of developing NODAT need to be prescribed the least diabetogenic immunosuppressant therapy. Herrero *et al.* (2003) identify an increased disposition to NODAT following transplantation when calcineurin inhibitors (cyclosporine A) are prescribed. The action of these drugs results in diminished insulin synthesis or release, due to islet cell toxicity and a decrease in peripheral insulin sensitivity. This in turn results in greater insulin resistance, which increases the insulin demand on the already struggling beta cells. A state of hyperinsulinaemia occurs that further exacerbates the insulin resistance, which increases other metabolic risk factors such as hypertension and hyperlipidaemia (Broom 2006).

Patients deemed at high risk, but who do not go on to develop NODAT in the preoperative phase, should continue to be screened postoperatively, as most cases develop within the first 3 months after transplantation (Sato *et al.* 2003). Ideally, patients should have a fasting plasma glucose level recorded every week for the first 4 weeks post-transplant, then again at 3, 6 and 12 months and annually thereafter. If a fasting plasma glucose level above 7 mmol/l is detected, then according to the World Health Organization guidelines (WHO 2006) a repeat fasting plasma blood glucose level should be recorded on a different day. If the result of this is above 7 mmol/l a diagnosis of diabetes is made and diabetes management instigated.

A fasting plasma of ≥6.1 mmol/ but <7.0 mmol/l indicates impaired fasting glycaemia and an oral glucose tolerance test may be required to determine whether or not diabetes has developed.

Conclusion

This chapter has considered the increasing link between diabetes and liver disease and demonstrated that, as the levels of obesity continue to rise worldwide, so do the number of people diagnosed with diabetes and liver disease.

NAFLD appears to be the main culprit and has a strong association with obesity and the metabolic syndrome, with insulin resistance being reported in almost all of the cases identified. Prevention and treatment for this has been discussed and includes the need to amend diet and lifestyle to achieve weight loss and increased insulin sensitivity. Treatment modalities to decrease the high levels of dyslipidaemia, often seen in these patients, have been identified, and the need to reduce the increased risk of cardiovascular disease these people exhibit has been highlighted.

HH, a different liver disease to NAFLD, has been emphasized and its association with the development of diabetes discussed. While the treatment and management of haemochromatosis is relatively simple and straightforward, it can have implications on the management of blood glucose levels. Suggestions on how blood glucose levels may be affected and how these can be dealt with effectively have been offered.

Finally, the care of a person with advanced liver disease and diabetes who is awaiting a liver transplant has been critically considered. Implications for practice and how the liver disease may affect diabetes control have been discussed with potential problem-solving solutions given. Awareness is also raised regarding the significant number of people who develop NODAT. By conducting a thorough assessment of the patient pre-transplant and identifying those as 'high risk' of developing diabetes it has been shown that treatment can be amended to reduce the overall risk.

Discharging the patient with diabetes from hospital

Aims of the chapter

This chapter will:

1. Consider the impact of the rising number of people being diagnosed with diabetes and its impact on the resources and cost of in-patient care.
2. Identify ways of reducing hospital admissions for people with diabetes via the recommendations of the National Service Framework (NSF) for Diabetes, Standard 8, focusing on medications and glycaemic targets.
3. Critically appraise and apply the partnership approach to care as advocated in Standard 3 of the NSF for Diabetes through the year of care project and care planning process.
4. Appraise the role structured education and information prescriptions can play in helping to reduce hospital admission rates.

As the prevalence of diabetes is set to rise significantly over the next 10 years or so, then the number of hospital admissions for diabetes-related complications will inevitably increase, which will have a knock-on effect of increasing in-patient costs. It is already known that, at any given time, between 6 and 16% of all hospital beds are occupied by someone with diabetes and that people with diabetes spend 1.1 million days in hospital each year, mainly to receive treatment to deal with the long-term complications of diabetes (ABPI/Diabetes UK 2006). The greatest impact on hospitalization rates is currently due to cardiovascular complications (Carral *et al.* 2003).

Olveira-Fuster *et al.* (2004) found that during 1999 the rate of admission to hospital was 145 per 1000 inhabitants for people with diabetes, compared with 70 admissions per 1000 inhabitants for individuals without diabetes. This shows that people with diabetes are more than twice as likely to experience hospitalization due to diabetes. Olveira-Fuster *et al.* (2004) also found that when they compared hospital admission per age group with those who do not have diabetes, the rate of admission for the under 15 year olds with diabetes was 468 per 1000, versus 45 admissions per 1000 inhabitants, which is a very significant difference. The 45–75-year-old group had the next highest admission rate of 230 admissions per 1000 population for people with diabetes, compared to only 88 admissions per 1000 population in those without.

These are quite staggering figures, which will impact heavily on healthcare budgets and resources. The study also highlighted that almost 60% of all hospital costs for in-patient care were due to chronic or acute disease related complications, particularly those related to cardiovascular disease, as mentioned. It is postulated that 75% of the excess costs were incurred by the 45–75-year-old age group with diabetes (Olveira-Fuster et al. 2004).

Although this study was conducted across Spanish hospitals, the rates of diabetes in Spain are similar to those seen in the UK and the results, which are comparable with studies in other countries, give confidence that the findings can be generalized. Also it can only be assumed that if the study were to be repeated today these figures would be even higher, based on the fact that disproportionately more people are now diagnosed with diabetes.

Not only are patients with diabetes more likely to be admitted to hospital, but they are also more likely to remain in hospital for a longer period of time when compared to their counterparts who do not have diabetes. The reasons for this are thought to be because of greater case severity (Carral et al. 2002), but there is also some thought that it may be due to less than optimal management and delivery of diabetes care. This is evidenced by many patients with diabetes reporting dissatisfaction with the quality of their diabetes in-patient care; there is often a lack of staff competency in diabetes management on non-specialist wards, and patients are not reviewed or managed by a specialist diabetes team. Patients also complain about the loss of control they experience regarding their diet, mealtimes, timing of oral medication and insulin injections (Bhattacharyya et al. 2000).

In attempts to address these problems and reduce bed occupancy, many acute trusts have set up a diabetes in-patient specialist service, in which patients admitted to a general ward can be referred to a diabetes specialist nurse or team for review and management advice. Experience of this has shown diabetes care to be improved, but the service is generally overstretched and healthcare professionals in non-specialist areas ideally need to take responsibility for ensuring that they have the basic competencies to provide appropriate care and management to patients with diabetes. The services of the specialist team could then be reserved for those patients who have more complex diabetes needs and as a result require a greater problem-solving and challenging approach to care.

As Sampson et al. (2006) point out, in the UK there is a drive to further reduce the bed occupancy by patients with chronic diseases such as diabetes. Most of this pressure has focused around reducing the admission rates of people with diabetes via improved medical management in primary care, rather than by reducing the length of stay in hospital. It is for these reasons that the healthcare professional working within secondary care needs to have an understanding of the care and management that can be provided within primary care and vice versa if a 'joined up' and 'seamless' approach to diabetes care is to be achieved.

National Service Framework

In attempts to improve the care and management of people with diabetes, and hopefully prevent the complications of diabetes from occurring or developing further and therefore reducing the number of people requiring hospitalization, the UK Department of Health in 2003 launched the National Service Framework (NSF) for Diabetes Delivery Strategy (Department of Health 2003). This set out a vision for diabetes services in England to be delivered by 2013. The aim of the NSF is to reduce the burden of diabetes in primary care, acute hospitals and community services and reduce the potentially devastating impact of the disease on individuals and their significant others. Similar documents have been produced for Scotland, Wales and Ireland.

The NSF identifies nine key areas in which diabetes care should be targeted, and sets out 12 standards for the prevention and management of diabetes. They also clearly highlight the active role people with diabetes will be encouraged to take on regarding the decisions made about their care (Table 9.1).

Standard 8

While all of the NSF standards can be applied to a number of different health care scenarios and a range of situations experienced by individuals with diabetes, Standard 8 specifically highlights the need for effective and timely care when the person is admitted to hospital. Within this standard comes the recommendation that people with diabetes should continue to be involved in the decisions regarding their care and the management of their diabetes during periods of hospitalization (Department of Health 2001). This is an area of healthcare that is generally lacking and there is a tendency for nurses and doctors to adopt a more medical approach and 'take over' the diabetes care when the patient is admitted to hospital. Unfortunately, in many instances the care and management given by the healthcare team to the person with diabetes is not always the most appropriate.

It must be recognized that up to 95% of the management of diabetes and the control of blood glucose levels is carried out by the patient, 24 hours each day, 7 days per week. The patient is the expert in how their body will react in certain situations and they should have been encouraged to develop their problem-solving skills to be able to react appropriately to differing blood glucose levels. Nobody knows their diabetes as well as the patient does, therefore the healthcare team needs to be able to provide the patient with the necessary tools, skills and equipment to be able to manage their diabetes control while in hospital. This will mean allowing the patient to monitor and chart their own blood glucose levels, give their own insulin at a time that coincides with meal times, adjust the amount of insulin they inject according to their blood glucose levels and be able to have access to snacks and high sugar foods in the event of a hypoglycaemic episode.

Table 9.1 National Service Framework (NSF) standards of care (Department of Health 2001).

Key area	Aim	Standards
Prevention of type 2 diabetes	To reduce the number of people who develop type 2 diabetes.	**Standard 1** The NHS will develop, implement and monitor strategies to reduce the risk of developing type 2 diabetes in the population as a whole and to reduce the inequalities in the risk of developing type 2 diabetes.
Identification of people with diabetes	To ensure that people with diabetes are identified as early as possible.	**Standard 2** The NHS will develop, implement and monitor strategies to identify people who do not know they have diabetes.
Empowering people with diabetes	To ensure that people with diabetes are empowered to enhance their personal control over the day-to-day management of their diabetes in a way that enables them to experience the best possible quality of life.	**Standard 3** All children, young people and adults with diabetes will receive a service that encourages partnership in decision making, supports them in managing their diabetes and helps them to adopt and maintain a healthy lifestyle. This will be reflected in an agreed and shared care plan in an appropriate format and language. Where appropriate, parents and carers should be fully engaged in this process.
Clinical care of adults with diabetes	To maximize the quality of life of all people with diabetes and to reduce their risk of developing the long-term complications of diabetes.	**Standard 4** All adults with diabetes will receive high-quality care throughout their lifetime, including support to optimize the control of their blood glucose, blood pressure and other risk factors for developing the complications of diabetes.
Clinical care of children and young people with diabetes	To ensure that the special needs of children and young people with diabetes are recognized and met, thereby ensuring that, when they enter adulthood, they are in the best of health and able to manage their own day-to-day diabetes care effectively.	**Standard 5** All children and young people with diabetes will receive consistently high-quality care and they, with their families and others involved in their day-to-day care, will be supported to optimize the control of their blood glucose and their physical, psychological, intellectual, educational and social development. **Standard 6** All young people with diabetes will experience a smooth transition of care from paediatric diabetes services to adult diabetes services, whether hospital or community based, either directly or via a young people's clinic. The transition will be organized in partnership with each individual and at an age appropriate to and agreed with them.

Management of diabetic emergencies	To minimize the impact on people with diabetes of the acute complications of diabetes.	**Standard 7** The NHS will develop, implement and monitor agreed protocols for rapid and effective treatment of diabetic emergencies by appropriately trained healthcare professionals. Protocols will include the management of acute complications and procedures to minimize the risk of recurrence.
Care of people with diabetes during admission to hospital	To ensure good-quality consistent care is provided for people with diabetes whenever they are admitted to hospital.	**Standard 8** All children, young people and adults with diabetes admitted to hospital, for whatever reason, will receive effective care of their diabetes. Wherever possible, they will continue to be involved in decisions concerning the management of their diabetes.
Diabetes and pregnancy	To achieve a good outcome and experience of pregnancy and childbirth for women with pre-existing diabetes and those who develop diabetes in pregnancy.	**Standard 9** The NHS will develop, implement and monitor policies that seek to empower and support women with pre-existing diabetes and those who develop diabetes during pregnancy to optimize the outcomes of their pregnancy.
Detection and management of long-term complications	To minimize the impact of the long-term complications of diabetes by early detection and effective treatment and by maximizing the quality of life of those who develop long-term complications.	**Standard 10** All young people and adults with diabetes will receive regular surveillance for the long-term complications of diabetes. **Standard 11** The NHS will develop, implement and monitor agreed protocols and systems of care to ensure that all people who develop long-term complications of diabetes receive timely, appropriate and effective investigation and treatment to reduce their risk of disability and premature death. **Standard 12** All people with diabetes requiring multi-agency support will receive integrated health and social care.

NHS, National Health Service.

Obviously, there are going to be situations within the ward and hospital environment when the patient is unable to maintain self-management of their blood glucose levels. In these cases the healthcare team will assume control, but only temporarily until the patient becomes self-caring again. It is also recognized that there are some people who are happy to surrender and delegate the control of their diabetes either while they are in hospital, or on a more permanent basis. In these situations it is important, prior to discharge home, that the patient is able and competent to recommence their blood glucose monitoring, record the results and act upon any abnormal readings that they may have.

Clearly, if costly hospital admissions for people with diabetes are to be minimized, effective tripartite communication needs to take place between the hospital, patient and general practitioner (GP). The GP needs to know in detail changes in management that have been implemented during hospitalization and the hospital needs to know how diabetes care is managed within the primary care setting to ensure that the most appropriate information is shared. The patient also needs to be fully aware of changes that have been made, the rationale for these changes and the potential effects on future management and decisions.

1. Medications

A survey by the Association of the British Pharmaceutical Industry (ABPI) and Diabetes UK (ABPI/Diabetes UK 2006) found that more than 33% of patients with diabetes did not appreciate that they had the condition for life and that 1 in 5 people with diabetes were not taking their medications as prescribed as they were not aware of the complications that can occur with poor glycaemic control.

Owing to the diversity and multitude of complications that can arise, many people with diabetes are prescribed a cocktail of different drugs, particularly if they develop kidney or cardiovascular disease. Polypharmacy is therefore a very common problem among people with diabetes, in that they are either not taking all of their prescribed medications, or they are taking them at inappropriate times. A period of hospitalization can compound these issues for different reasons. First, the patient who is compliant in taking their medications has developed a systematic and foolproof system at home to ensure that the medications are taken at the correct times of the day; however, during admission to hospital, administration of medicines is generally done by the nursing staff, therefore stripping the patient of their autonomy. Even if the medications remain exactly the same on discharge home, the patient may have forgotten their routine, which can lead to difficulties with compliance.

More often than not, a period of hospitalization will result in changes being made to the medications people with diabetes are prescribed. In these scenarios it is vitally important that time is taken prior to discharge home to explain clearly to the patient exactly the action and use of each of the prescribed medications, any changes in dose and the optimum times of day in which to take the tablets and/or insulin. Prior to discharge, the healthcare professional needs to be satisfied that the patient is still able to give themselves their insulin injections or have a back-up system to enable this to happen. Additionally, patients need to have the mental and physical capacity to be able to administer their prescribed oral medications at the required time of day. Failure to address these basic principles could result in readmission to hospital within a very short space of time.

It also needs to be reinforced that only a limited supply of each of the tablets is given on discharge home, therefore the patient will need to ensure that they obtain further supplies via their GP. Each year a significant number of people do not continue their prescribed medication once they have taken what they were sent home with, as they do not appreciate that they need to keep taking the tablets until told otherwise and, for example, should be informed that their prescription is different from taking a finite course of antibiotics.

The prescribing GP also needs to be fully informed of the changes in medication. If doses of oral medications have been changed, these need to be communicated; a comprehensive list of the new medications to be prescribed should be given. In cases where insulin has been altered, the GP needs to be informed of what insulin is now being taken, at what time of day it is to be taken, the number of units in each dose and the type of insulin pen and needles being used to administer the insulin. The GP will also need to know the correct replacement insulin vial for the insulin pen or whether the patient is using a prefilled, disposable pen. Patients will also need to be informed of how the pen works if it is new to them, and whether or not it is a reusable one. Additionally, patients who are new to taking insulin will need to be prescribed a sharps' disposal box and informed of how to dispose of sharps safely.

Patients and their GPs need to be aware that the dose of medications used to lower blood glucose levels will need to be reviewed following discharge from hospital. This is due to the potential effect that illness and hospitalization may have on the blood glucose levels resulting from an increase in pain, stress, infection, etc. and subsequent adrenaline release. Once this stress response subsides, the doses of any insulin or oral antidiabetes medications may need to be reduced to prevent hypoglycaemia. Patients should also be encouraged to monitor their blood glucose levels more frequently for a period of time following discharge home to observe for these changes.

2. Glycaemic control targets at home

When a person with diabetes is admitted to hospital for a period of time, due to an acute or chronic illness, there may be times when they are very unwell and blood glucose levels may be higher than normally expected. As mentioned previously, this may be due to the stress response and increased secretion of adrenaline or due to such factors as infection. Upon discharge from hospital the patient needs to be made fully aware that, now they have overcome the illness and are fit enough to return home, they should endeavour to achieve blood glucose levels within the target range of 4–7 mmol/l. This is particularly important if the person has a wound that requires further healing, as high blood glucose levels can delay or prevent the natural healing process.

If patients are given new equipment such as blood glucose monitoring machines when they are in hospital, this information will also be required by the GP to ensure that the correct testing strips for the new machine are prescribed in the future. In this instance, the patient also needs to be discharged with an adequate supply of testing strips so that they can monitor their blood glucose levels until the GP can generate a new prescription.

Inevitably, there will be some patients who will have difficulties maintaining their blood glucose levels within normal parameters following discharge from hospital, and their needs are more complex. Furthermore, due to the nature of diabetes, many may be experiencing difficulties with co-morbidities. In these instances, a referral to the community matron may be appropriate to ensure the diabetes is managed appropriately and to help prevent further complications from arising.

Standard 3

The diabetes NSF is committed to people taking a more active role in their diabetes management and being part of the decision making process. As David Levy, a consultant diabetologist, points out: 'there is a need to educate healthcare professionals and patients alike to look ahead, rather than just focusing on short-term achievements such as reducing blood sugar levels' (ABPI/DUK 2006).

1. Care planning

Standard 3 of the NSF stipulates the production of an agreed care plan that takes a holistic view of the individual person with diabetes. Within the care plan, the patient and, where appropriate, parents and carers will have had the opportunity to provide input on the decisions made. The thinking behind this approach is based on the notion that people do not like to be told what to do, therefore if the goals of care are generated and agreed by the patient it is more likely that they will be achieved. Furthermore, it is thought that patients will become more knowledgeable about their condition and the required management strategies (National Diabetes Support Team 2008). It could also have a positive impact on patient referrals, as only the motivated and committed patients would be referred to a dietitian for instance as they would have highlighted a need for this in their care plan. This could reduce the number of non-attendees to the clinic/consultation and increase the overall clinic outcomes when they are audited.

The potential difficulties with this approach are based on findings published in The Diabetes Information Jigsaw (ABPI/Diabetes UK 2006). This report found that over half of people with diabetes do not find it easy to ask questions about their treatments and management as they feel that not enough time is allocated during their consultation to answer all of their queries. They were also reluctant to ask questions as their nurse or doctor always appeared to be too busy. However, what is not evident in the report is the notion that not all people have a good understanding of diabetes and its management and therefore do not know what questions to ask.

There are also a number of implications of implementing the care planning approach for healthcare professionals. They will need to learn to adopt a very different approach to their consultations, allowing a more questioning and open avenue. They will need to understand how a care planning approach differs from an acute model of care and be committed to the principles of working in partnership with people with diabetes. This may create quite a challenge for some healthcare professionals and could require modification of their current role and responsibilities.

Healthcare practitioners will also need to develop a very different 'philosophy' of diabetes care. The patient is the one who determines the targets and goals to be met, but may not be congruent with the current evidence base. For example, current guidelines advocate a haemoglobin A1c (HbA1c) result of between 6.5 and 7.5% in order to significantly reduce complications. In order to achieve this, the patient needs to keep their blood glucose levels with the 4–7 mmol/l range for a significant portion of each day. However, a person with an HbA1c of 10% may decide that they are happy with their current diabetes control and do not want to try and reduce their blood glucose levels any further, despite being fully aware of the potentially serious ramifications of their decision. Within the care planning approach the healthcare practitioner would have to accept this patient's decision, knowing that it could lead to more serious and costly complications in the future. Additionally, it would mean that additional services would not be commissioned as the patient would not deem them necessary.

This is a difficult concept, as healthcare professionals know that reducing the costs associated with admission to hospital requires aggressive control by primary healthcare teams in the prevention of complications. Waiting until the person has developed the complications and is therefore going to require hospital management is like 'closing the stable door once the horse has bolted'. Management of obesity, blood pressure and dyslipidaemia is required and the treatment for the overall control of the diabetes needs to be intensified to avoid complications and hospital admission.

2. Year of care
Currently, people with diabetes in the community are provided with a standard care package that includes an annual review to assess overall diabetes control and to test and screen for the development of any diabetes-related complications. The information from this annual review is then fed into the Quality Outcomes Framework (2006/07), which most GPs have signed up to. This is a tick box process in which biomedical variables such as HbA1c, blood pressure and foot sensation are measured and recorded. It is structured to identify where individual general practices have achieved the set quality indicators, and they are then awarded points that are attached to specific funding. The more points that are awarded, the higher the level of funding received. This yields incentives to deliver good patient care and gives money to reinvest into services provided by the practice.

The 'year of care' concept has been developed by Professor Pieter Degeling at the Centre for Clinical Management Development, University of Durham. He would like to see patients being provided with a more holistic review of care, in which the patient is placed firmly in the centre. Their individual needs and requirements to enable them to deal with, and control, their diabetes for the next year would be discussed, agreed and then documented in a care plan. The care plan would identify if the patient is likely to require any additional services such as diet and nutrition or podiatry in the forthcoming year; if so, these can then be costed. Surgeries within each primary care trust would then combine the information from all the individual care plans to determine what services are required and to what extent; from this, effective commissioning of services could be achieved. For these reasons, it is envisaged that the year of care concept is ideally suited to a UK National Health Service (NHS) based in primary care providing comprehensive diabetes services. However, for this approach to be successful, a complete overhaul of the current Quality and Outcomes Framework would be required.

While this approach is a positive step in providing holistic care that the patient has agreed, and is helpful in providing a framework for clinical governance and for auditing standards of care, it fails to deal with what happens in the event that a person with diabetes requires hospitalization and as a result their care and management is altered significantly. This highlights the complex nature of long-term conditions like diabetes and raises questions on how emergency care will be funded if the individual budget for the year has already been allocated or exceeded.

To ensure that the person receives the right care at the right time, it would seem more appropriate for the care plan to be owned by the patient and amended by the hospital or community healthcare team as their condition changes. This would also help to bring together more closely those in primary, specialist and community care to provide a joined-up and seamless approach to care of the person with diabetes. Additionally, people with diabetes need to be kept fully informed of the new processes and structures, their rights, entitlements and how an individual budget system will work for them.

Structured education

In order for care planning and the year of care concept to be accepted and utilized effectively in practice, people with diabetes will need to have access to high-quality information and education, both in the hospital and after discharge home. This should take the form of a planned, life-long process, commencing at the point of diagnosis and continuing as an essential component of diabetes care and management thereafter.

The National Institute for Health and Clinical Excellence (NICE) Health Technology Appraisal Guidance (NICE 2003) defines structured education as 'a planned and graded programme that is comprehensive in scope, flexible in content, responsive to an individual's clinical and psychological needs and adaptable to his or her educational and cultural background'. The overall aim of education is to provide people with diabetes with the knowledge, skills, tools and confidence that will enable them to take an increasingly active role in the effective self-management of their condition. It is believed that if patients are more pro-active in their diabetes management, the risk of developing complications will be lessened, resulting in a reduced need to be admitted to hospital, thus reducing hospital bed occupancy.

All healthcare professionals working with primary or secondary care can, and should be encouraged to, provide structured education, but the NICE Health Technology Appraisal (NICE 2003) on patient education found that while most patients were offered education, this differed significantly between providers in terms of length, content and quality. In attempts to standardize patient education and ensure that it fulfils the NICE requirements, the Patient Education Working Group agreed a set of quality standards and key criteria which all education programmes should meet. The key criteria state that education programmes should:

- have a structured, written curriculum,
- have trained educators,
- be quality assured,
- be audited.

Following on from these guidelines, the NICE Health Technology Appraisal Guidance (NICE 2003) recommend that structured patient education models should consider a number of key issues if they are to achieve maximum learning and be cost effective. The recommendations include:

- Educational interventions should consider the current evidence base on the principles and theories of adult learning.
- Education should be provided to groups of people with diabetes by an appropriately trained multidisciplinary team.
- The delivery of the sessions should be considered to ensure maximum accessibility by a broad range of people from a variety of cultural and ethnic backgrounds. Access to those with a disability also needs to be addressed.
- Given the different learning styles of individuals, the educational programmes should employ a variety of different approaches and teaching methods to ensure that all members of the group engage with the taught content and consequently enhance their learning.

Time, energy and commitment are therefore required from healthcare professionals if they want to deliver high-quality patient education.

Education for the healthcare professional also needs to be given serious consideration, as having a working knowledge of diabetes and its management and complications is not enough. Healthcare professionals need to learn the theory and practice of teaching and learning so that differing levels of education within the group are addressed, the individual learning needs of the group are met via a variety of different teaching strategies and resources, and any barriers to education and learning are broken down effectively.

National programmes

There are currently three main national group education programmes for adults with diabetes in the UK that meet the key criteria for structured education. They are: (1) dose adjustment for normal eating (DAFNE); (2) diabetes education and self-management for ongoing and newly diagnosed (DESMOND); and (3) the diabetes X-PERT programme. These courses can be bought and implemented at a local level, but there are a number of other courses that are becoming available nationally. Additionally, there are a number of local adult education groups who are developing their education programmes to meet the current criteria for structured education (Valerkou 2006). Therefore, in providing structured education, healthcare professionals need to consider what is currently available, whether it meets the specific needs of their client group, and the cost of delivering it compared to devising and delivering their own education package that also meets the required criteria.

Dose Adjustment For Normal Eating (DAFNE)

DAFNE is a skills-based education programme aimed at adults with type 1 diabetes. It has been developed around the evidence presented by the Diabetes Control and Complications Trial Research Group (DCCT) (1993), which identified that keeping blood glucose levels as close to normal limits as possible can considerably reduce the risk of microvascular complications of diabetes. However, in utilizing the findings of the DCCT, the DAFNE Collaborative (2003) acknowledged potential difficulties that had to be borne in mind. They recognized that only a few patients aim for near-normal blood glucose levels and a large proportion of people with diabetes do not test their blood glucose levels or act on the results. Additionally, current insulin regimens as mentioned in Chapter 2 are not sophisticated enough to be able to mimic the pulsing action of the healthy pancreas and thus inhibit the person's ability to control blood glucose levels adequately.

Despite these difficulties, it was believed by the group that subcutaneous insulin could control blood glucose levels within normal parameters by integrating a number of different principles. During a visit to the World Health Organization (WHO) Collaborating Centre for Diabetes in Düsseldorf, the DAFNE group observed a 5-day structured training programme for patients in intensive insulin therapy and self-management. Subsequent research following attendance at the educational programme found that people with type 1 diabetes were able to achieve significant reductions in HbA1c levels, which were maintained over time. From this visit, the DAFNE group believed that type 1 diabetes could be managed by insulin replacement as needed, and not by dietary manipulation to fit in with set amounts of prescribed insulin.

A 5-day course was developed that aimed to provide people with the skills necessary to enable them to replace insulin by matching it to the amount of carbohydrate in each meal. People were taught how to count grams of carbohydrate, and were advised that they could eat whatever they wanted and no longer needed to heed dietary restrictions. However, there was the premise that people should follow the principles for healthy eating and that being allowed a free diet should not be translated into being able to have a high-calorie, fat-laden diet. They were also taught, using adult education principles, the action of insulin and given the knowledge and confidence to be able to adjust insulin doses to meet their specific requirements.

Put simply, people are commenced on a four times per day basal/bolus insulin regimen, if not already on this, and taught the skills of being able to calculate how much carbohydrate is in the meal they are about to eat. This may be a meal they have cooked themselves, or it may be in a restaurant, and they will need to take into consideration the carbohydrate content of each course and any drinks taken at the same time. Based upon their own personally calculated insulin to carbohydrate ratio, they will calculate how much insulin is needed to control blood glucose levels following ingestion of that particular meal. They are also taught how to give 'correction' doses of insulin if their blood glucose levels are higher than expected preprandially, thus ensuring a much closer match between insulin and carbohydrate requirements and resulting in improved blood glucose control.

Research was conducted into the efficacy of the education course (DAFNE Study Group 2002); after 6 months, those who had attended the DAFNE training programme had experienced a fall in HbA1c of 1% compared to the control group, with no increase in the risk of hypoglycaemia. At 1 year, glycaemic control had deteriorated slightly but there still remained a 0.5% reduction in HbA1c.

In March 2002 the Expert Patient Programme provided a grant of £500 000 to the DAFNE project to enable seven new centres to be trained to provide DAFNE courses (DAFNE Collaborative 2003). Since then DAFNE has continued to grow substantially, with more and more centres nationwide now delivering the programme. Reviews and evaluations from patients have been positive. Comments from people who have undertaken the course include, 'I've taken control of a condition that had previously controlled me,' and 'Thank you for this opportunity and for giving me my life back' (DAFNE Collaborative 2003).

Diabetes Education and Self-management for Ongoing and Newly Diagnosed (DESMOND)

This is another structured group education programme for adults newly diagnosed with type 2 diabetes. This education programme has been carefully designed and evaluated using the UK Medical Research Council's framework for complex interventions and has a theoretical and philosophical base. It also meets the standards outlined in the NSF for Diabetes and by NICE. The educational intervention was devised as a group education programme that would be delivered in a community setting and integrated into routine care (Davies *et al.* 2008). It is delivered by healthcare professionals who have received formal training and are subject to a quality assurance mechanism that ensures consistency of delivery.

However, it could be argued that while quality and consistency of the educational provision is paramount, there also needs to be some flexibility in the delivery of the curriculum. Not every group being taught has the same characteristics, educational levels, cultural and religious beliefs, and learning styles; all differ from group to group and these need to be considered and the appropriate teaching and facilitating strategies applied. Additionally, all healthcare professionals are unique and need to be able to bring to the programme their own style of teaching in order for it to be effective and worthwhile.

The DESMOND programme began to be developed in 2003 and is made up of 6 hours of group sessions, delivered in the community to a maximum of 10 people newly diagnosed with type 2 diabetes. It aims to support people in being able to identify their own health needs and be able to respond to them accordingly by setting their own behavioural goals. This sits very well with the proposed year of care (Diabetes UK 2008) and care-planning approach where it is envisaged that by the individual being able to recognize their own health risks this may help the person to become more motivated and take a pro-active role in the management of their diabetes control.

Following the success of the programme for people with newly diagnosed diabetes, the DESMOND team has now completed and made available a foundation programme for people with established diabetes, and a version of this is culturally appropriate for the South Asian community.

More recently in a large randomized control trial involving 207 general practices from 13 sites in England and Scotland, Davies *et al.* (2008) sought to determine the effectiveness of DESMOND on biomedical, psychosocial and lifestyle measures in people with newly diagnosed type 2 diabetes. In seeking these data, the trial had three important functions: (1) to evaluate the intervention itself and its level of generalizability; (2) to assess the effectiveness of providing structured group education at diagnosis; and (3) to show at what point any benefits of education begin to diminish (Davies *et al.* 2008).

The sample was divided into two groups: an intervention arm where the participants attended the DESMOND programme and a control group. The results are interesting as the main outcomes of HbA1c and quality of life did not differ significantly between the two groups; however, the DESMOND intervention group improved weight loss, rates of smoking cessation, beliefs about illness and self-reported depression. Dinneen (2008), a member of the DAFNE Collaborative, attempts to justify these findings by explaining that any improvement in metabolic control is often seen shortly after diagnosis so that any effect of structured education may have been masked. This is accepted, but participants in the Davies *et al.* (2008) group were recruited within only 12 weeks of diagnosis. Dinneen (2008) also suggests that participation in DESMOND requires the participants to set their own personal health goals and therefore they may have purposely chosen goals such as smoking cessation and/or weight loss over glycaemic control. This is feasible and serves to highlight a limitation of the study and flaw in the original study design.

Qualitative feedback on the DESMOND programme has been obtained from those attending the programme and comments include 'for the first time in years I feel better, I eat properly, I swim everyday, I walk approximately 40 km each week, I have gone from 97.5 kilos to 82.5 kilos. Having diabetes has improved my life.'

Diabetes X-PERT programme

The X-PERT programme is a 6-week structured education programme initially for people with type 2 diabetes, which is based upon the theories of patient empowerment, patient-centred care and activation. It also meets the key criteria to fulfil NICE guidance as well as embracing the philosophy underpinning the year of care and care planning in diabetes. The programme is currently being implemented throughout the UK and Ireland and has been adapted for children, adolescents, young adults and adults with type 1 diabetes.

A study by Deakin *et al.* (2006) set out to test the hypothesis 'Primary care delivery of the patient-centred, structured diabetes education programme X-PERT for adults with type 2 diabetes, based on theories of patient empowerment and discovery learning, develops skills and confidence leading to increased diabetes self-management and sustained improvements in clinical, lifestyle and psychosocial outcomes'. In this study, 314 participants were randomized to an intervention or control group. As far as possible blind allocation was carried out and the participants were unsure of which group they had been allocated. Members of the intervention group were invited to attend the X-PERT programme, which involved the 6-weekly education sessions, whereas the control group were given routine care and a prearranged individual appointment with a dietitian, practice nurse and GP. Baseline assessments of HbA1c, blood pressure, cholesterol, weight, body mass index (BMI), body fat % and waist size were carried out at the start of the research, and were repeated again at 14 months (Deakin *et al.* 2006).

Previous studies have shown that in the first 6 months following educational input, people with diabetes are still able to recall knowledge of what they have learned and adhere to dietary habits and glycaemic control (Norris *et al.* 2001). However, meta-analysis has shown that the benefits of education and self management on HbA1c begin to fall between 1 and 3 months after the intervention (Norris *et al.* 2002). Results from the longer term study by Deakin *et al.* (2006) showed that the participants in the X-PERT group had a greater reduction in HbA1c compared with the control group (0.6% versus 0.1%). Those who attended the X-PERT group also showed greater reductions in total cholesterol, body weight, BMI and waist circumference when compared with the control group. There was no statistically significant difference between the groups in relation to blood pressure, high-density lipoprotein (HDL), low-density lipoprotein (LDL) or triglycerides (Deakin *et al.* 2006). The findings of this study are particularly significant to the management and care of people with diabetes due to the demonstrated longer-term effects of the education programme.

General patient education prior to discharge from hospital

Discharging the patient with diabetes home from hospital will only be effective and the risk of readmission reduced if the healthcare professional is confident that the patient fully understands his or her condition and knows how to manage it themselves. The healthcare professional responsible for discharging a person who has been newly diagnosed with diabetes needs to ensure that they have given the patient as much information as possible to ensure that they are kept safe on discharge home and that referrals are in place for the person to attend the most appropriate diabetes education programme. Likewise, a person with long-standing diabetes may not have the most up-to-date knowledge and skills for effective self-management and may also benefit from attending a structured education course.

Information prescription

Information prescription is a new concept in diabetes care suggested by ABPI/ Diabetes UK (2006) as a step towards achieving Standard 3 of the NSF for diabetes. In encouraging a partnership approach to care and decision making and supporting patients to become self-managing of their diabetes, an information prescription could be provided. ABPI/Diabetes UK (2006) envisage that this would be most beneficial given by the healthcare professional at the time of the consultation and could be tailored to meet the individual's specific learning needs. After discussing with the person their concerns, fears, goals and their understanding of the diagnosis and treatment the healthcare professional could direct them to the most appropriate sources of further information and support.

The type of information used could include booklets, magazines, books, articles, posters and human resources, such as an appointment with the dietitian, could potentially link in with the already mentioned care planning approach. Sources on the internet would also be included once they had been 'approved' as appropriate by the prescribing healthcare professional. This would enable the patient and the healthcare professional to feel confident in the quality and accuracy of the information provided.

Information prescriptions could also be used effectively during hospitalization and on discharge home. The clinical area may have copies of information that can be loaned or given to the patient on an individual basis according to need. On discharge home, the patient will then be given a list of other information resources that they would be advised to follow up on.

Prescribing information for patients has to be done on an individual basis in order for it to be successful. Just giving the patient a 'reading list' will not necessarily meet their specific requirements; consideration also needs to be given to the person's cultural and religious beliefs as well as their educational level and whether they are computer literate and have access to the worldwide web. If used carefully and not abused, information prescriptions should improve the efficiency of consultations and the care and management provided. Also, matching the information to the particular patient will enable more effective informed consent.

Table 9.2 Checklist for discharging the person with diabetes from hospital.

Patient name:
Date of birth:
Hospital number:
General practitioner:

Discharge item	Applicable YES/NO	General practitioner/ community nurse informed (✓)	Patient/ significant other informed (✓)	Changes/ details
1 Blood glucose monitoring				
a Patient required to blood glucose monitor				
b Times of day when to blood glucose monitor identified				
	Patient able to act upon abnormal blood glucose readings			
c Blood glucose meter changed				
d Testing strips changed				
2 Medication				
a Information given on medications prescribed on discharge from hospital				
b Explanation given to patient on action and side-effects of prescribed medications				
c Doses of prescribed medications have been changed				
d Patient needs to order a repeat prescription for medications prescribed on discharge home				
e Patient understands and is able to take medications at prescribed times				
f Changes made to insulin regimen				
g New insulin regimen documented and communicated				
h New insulin pen prescribed				
i New insulin pen needles prescribed				
j Replacement insulin vial has been changed				
k Patient able to use insulin pen competently				
l Need to review medication postdischarge				

Continued

Table 9.2 Continued

Patient name:
Date of birth:
Hospital number:
General practitioner:

Discharge item	Applicable YES/NO	General practitioner/ community nurse informed (✓)	Patient/ significant other informed (✓)	Changes/ details
3 Referrals				
a Patient goals discussed				
b Community matron				
c Dietitian				
d Podiatry				
e Structured education				
f Information prescription				
4 Biochemical markers				
a Haemoglobin A1c (HbA1c)				
b Blood glucose				
c Blood pressure				
d Total cholesterol				
e High-density lipoprotein (HDL)				
f Low-density lipoprotein (LDL)				
g Triglycerides				
h Urea and electrolytes				
i Creatinine				
j				
k				
l				
m				
n				

Specific instructions/details:

Checklist for discharging the person with diabetes from hospital

Table 9.2 provides a simple checklist to facilitate the transition for the patient from hospital back to home and to ensure that the patient and their GP/community nurse are fully informed of the decisions made while the patient has been in hospital and of the follow-up care that is required. It can also serve as a communication tool between primary and secondary care and facilitate the referral process to other members of the multidisciplinary team.

Conclusion

In conclusion, the discharge from hospital needs to be timely, smooth and efficient. Priority of care is needed to ensure that diabetes specialists and primary care teams collaborate in the development of strategies and the management of care to prevent diabetes complications from arising. Multiprofessional teams across all healthcare sectors need to work together to ensure that people with diabetes are able to make informed decisions and are empowered and supported to take control of their diabetes so that they are able to achieve a good quality of life while living with a long-term condition.

This chapter has focused primarily on the impact that the rising number of people being diagnosed with diabetes is having on the current resources and cost of inpatient care. Using the NSF for Diabetes as a tool, Standards 3 and 8 have been considered as ways of reducing the diabetes burden on hospital beds.

Some of the common pitfalls that patients and healthcare practitioners have to deal with have been discussed, including compliance with medications, and the changing glycaemic targets during hospitalization and on discharge home.

Currently, a main focus of diabetes care is the need for patients to become more knowledgeable and skilled at being able to make decisions about their own care and to be able to effectively problem solve different situations in order to achieve and maintain good glycaemic control. To this end, the year of care project and a care-planning approach to diabetes have been discussed and the link highlighted between these and the role of structured education and information prescription.

References

ABPI/Diabetes UK (2006) Ask about medicines. Diabetes Medicines Information Survey. http://www.abpi.org.uk/%2Fpublications%2Fpdfs%2Fdiabetes_jigsaw.pdf (accessed 15 July 2008).

Ahmed, B. (2004) Pharmacology of insulin. *Diabetes and Vascular Disease*, **4**, 10–13.

Akerblom, H.K., Vaarala, O., Hyoty, H., Ilanen, J. and Knip, M. (2002) Environmental factors in the etiology of type 1 diabetes. *American Journal of Medical Genetics*, **115**, 18–29.

Albarran, N.B., Ballesteros, M.N., Morales, G.G. and Ortega, M.I. (2006) Dietary behaviour and type 2 diabetes care. *Patient Education and Counselling*, **61**, 191–9.

Alberti, K.G.M.M. and Thomas, D.J.B. (1979) The management of diabetes during surgery. *British Journal of Anaesthesia*, **51**, 693–710.

Alberti, K.G.M.M., Simmet, P. and Shaw, J. (2005) The metabolic syndrome – a new worldwide definition. *The Lancet*, **366**, 1059–62.

American Diabetes Association (2003) Report of the Expert Committee on the Diagnosis and Classification of Diabetes Mellitus. *Diabetes Care*, **26**, S5–20.

American Diabetes Association (2004a) Hypertension management in adults with diabetes. *Diabetes Care*, **27**, S65–7.

American Diabetes Association (2004b) Nephropathy in diabetes (position statement). *Diabetes Care*, **27** (Suppl.1), S79–83.

American Diabetes Association (2005a) Tests of glycaemia in diabetes. *Diabetes Care*, **27**, S91–3.

American Diabetes Association (2005b) Standards of medical care in diabetes. *Diabetes Care*, **38**, S4–36.

American Diabetes Association (2006) Diagnosis and classification of diabetes mellitus. *Diabetes Care*, **29**, S43–8.

Angulo, P. (2002) Non-alcoholic fatty liver disease. *New England Journal of Medicine*, **346**, 1221–31.

Angulo, P., Keach, J.C., Batts, K.P. and Lindor, K.D. (1999) Independent predictors of liver fibrosis in patients with nonalcoholic steatohepatitis. *Heptology*, **30**, 1356–62.

Antonelli, A., Ferrari, S.M., Ferri, C., *et al.* (2005) Hepatitis C virus infection. *Diabetes Care*, **28**, 2548–50.

Arner, P. (2005) Insulin resistance in type 2 diabetes – role of the adipokines. *Current Molecular Medicine*, **5**, 333–9.

Aschner, P., Kipnes, M., Lunceford, J., Mickel, C., Davies, M. and Williams-Hermann, D. (2006) Sitagliptin monotherapy improved glycaemic control in the fasting and post-prandial states and beta-cell function after 24 weeks in patients with type 2 diabetes (T2DM). *Diabetes*, **55**, (Suppl. 1), 462, (abstract 1995-PO).

Astrup, A. (2003) Is there any conclusive evidence that exercise alone reduces glucose intolerance? *The British Journal of Diabetes and Vascular Disease*, **3**, (Suppl. 1), S18–23.

Bäckman, L.A. (2004) Post-transplant diabetes mellitus: the last 10 years with tacrolimus. *Nephrology Dialysis Transplantation*, **19**, (Suppl. 6), vi13–vi16.

Bailey, C.J. and Feher, M.D. (2004) *Therapies for Diabetes*. Sherborne Gibbs, Birmingham.

Bazzano, L.A., Li, T.Y., Joshipura, K.J. and Hu, F.B. (2008) Intake of fruit, vegetables and fruit juices and risk of diabetes in women. *Diabetes Care*, **31**, 1311–17.

Belch, J., Stansby, G., Shearman, C., *et al.* (2007) Peripheral arterial disease – a cardio-vascular time bomb. *The British Journal of Diabetes and Vascular Disease*, **7**, 236–9.

Bhattacharyya, A., Christodoulides, C., Kaushal, K., New, J.P. and Young, R.J. (2000) Inpatient management of diabetes mellitus and patient satisfaction. *Diabetic Medicine*, **19**, 412–16.

Bleyer, A.J., Sedor, J.R., Freedman, B.I., *et al.* (2008) Risk factors for the development and progression of diabetic kidney disease and treatment patterns among diabetic siblings of patients with diabetic kidney disease. *American Journal of Kidney Disease*, **51**, 29–37.

Bloomgarden, Z.T. (2007) Diabetic neuropathy. *Diabetes Care*, **30**, 1027–32.

Bonifacio, E., Hummelm M., Walter, M., Schmid, S. and Ziegler, A.G. (2004) IDDM and multiple family history of Type 1 diabetes combine to identify neonates at high risk for type 1 diabetes. *Diabetes Care*, **27**, 2695–700.

Bosi, E., Conti, M., Vermigli, C., *et al.* (2005) Effectiveness of frequency-modulated electromagnetic neural stimulation in the treatment of painful diabetic neuropathy. *Diabetologia*, **48**, 817–23.

Boulton, A.J.M., Gries, F.A. and Jervell, J.A. (1998) Guidelines for the diagnosis and outpatient management diabetic peripheral neuropathy. *Diabetic Medicine*, **15**, 508–14.

Boulton, A.J.M., Kirsner, R.S. and Viliekyte, L. (2004) Neuropathic diabetic foot ulcers. *New England Journal of Medicine*, **351**, 48–55.

Boulton, A.J.M., Vinik, A.I., Arezzo, J.C., *et al.* (2005) Diabetic neuropathies. *Diabetes Care*, **28**, 956–62.

British National Formulary (2008) http://www.bnf.org/bnf/ (accessed 29 September 2008).

British Society for Haematology (2000) Genetic haemochromatosis. http://www.bcshguidelines.com (accessed 2 May 2008).

Brook, C.G. and Marshall, N.J. (2001) *Essential Endocrinology*. Blackwell Science, Oxford.

Broom, I. (2006) Thinking about abdominal obesity and cardiovascular risk. *The British Journal of Diabetes and Vascular Disease*, **6**, 58–61.

Bugianesi, E., Gentilcore, E., Manini, R., *et al.* (2005) A randomized controlled trial of metformin versus vitamin E or prescriptive diet in nonalcoholic fatty liver disease. *American Journal of Gastroenterology*, **100**, 1082–90.

Campbell, I.W. and Day, C. (2007) Sitagliptin – enhancing incretin action. *The British Journal of Diabetes and Vascular Disease*, **7**, 134–9.

Carr, D.B., Utzschneider, K.M., Hull, R.L., *et al.* (2004) Intra-abdominal fat is a major determinant of the National Cholesterol Education Program Adult Treatment Panel III criteria for the metabolic syndrome. *Diabetes*, **53**, 2087–94.

Carral, F., Olveira, G., Sala, J., Garcia, L., Sillero, A. and Aguilar, M. (2002) Care resource utilization and direct costs incurred by people with diabetes in a Spanish hospital. *Diabetes Research and Clinical Practice*, **56**, 27–34.

Carral, F., Aguilar, M., Oliveira, G., Mangas, A., Domenech, I. and Torres, I. (2003) Increased hospital expenditures in diabetic patients hospitalized for cardiovascular diseases. *Journal of Diabetes and its Complications*, **17**, 331–6.

Centre for Drug Evaluation and Research (1999). Approval package: Avandia (rosiglitazone maleate) tablets. Company: Smith Kline Beecham Pharmaceuticals. Application no. 21–071. Approval date: 5/25/1999. http://www.fda.gov/cder/foi/nda/99/21071_Avandia.htm (accessed 21 July 2007).

Chalasani, N., Aljadhey, H., Kesterson, J., Murray, M.D. and Hall, S.D. (2004) Patients with elevated liver enzymes are not at higher risk for statin hepatotoxicity. *Gastroenterology*, **126**, 1287–92.

Chan, W. (2003) *Food and Diet Counter*. Hamlyn, London.

Clayton, M. and Holt, P. (2006) Hereditary haemochromatosis and diabetes – implications for practice. *Gastrointestinal Nursing*, **4**, 22–6.

Clements, G.B., Galbraith, D.N. and Taylor, K.W. (1995) Coxsackie B virus infection and onset of childhood diabetes. *The Lancet*, **346**, 221–3.

Colhoun, H.M., Betteridge, D.J., Durrington, P.N., *et al.* (2004) Primary prevention of cardiovascular disease with atorvastatin in type 2 diabetes in the Collaborative Atorvastatin Diabetes Study (CARDS): multicentre randomised placebo-controlled trial. *The Lancet*, **364**, 685–96.

Colombani, P.C. (2004) Glycaemic index and load – dynamic dietary guidelines in the context of diseases. *Physiology and Behavior*, **83**, 603–10.

Confidential Enquiry into Maternal and Child Health (2007) http://www.cemach.org.uk (accessed 25 July 2007).

Conway, B., Fried, L. and Orchard, T. (2008) Haemoglobin and overt nephropathy complications in type 1 diabetes. *Annals of Epidemiology*, **18**, 147–55.

Cooper, M.E. (1998) Pathogenesis, prevention, and treatment of diabetic nephropathy. *The Lancet*, **352**, 213–19.

Cowburn, C. (2004) Preventing type 2 diabetes by preventing obesity: what do population-based approaches offer? *Obesity in Practice*, **6**, 13–15.

Cummings, J., Mineo, K., Levy, R. and Josephson, R.A. (1999) A review of the DIGAMI study: intensive insulin therapy during and after myocardial infarctions in diabetic patients. *Diabetes Spectrum*, **12**, 84–8.

DAFNE Collaborative (2003) DAFNE Collaborative: the roll-out experience. http://www. dafne.uk.com/downloads.DoH%20report.pdf (accessed 14 July 2008).

DAFNE Study Group (2002) Training in flexible, intensive insulin management to enable dietary freedom in people with type 1 diabetes: dose adjustment for normal eating (DAFNE) randomised controlled trial. *British Medical Journal*, **325**, 746.

Davies, M.J., Heller, S., Skinner, T.C., *et al.* (2008) Effectiveness of the diabetes education and self management for ongoing and newly diagnosed (DESMOND) programme for people with newly diagnosed type 2 diabetes: cluster randomised controlled trial. *British Medical Journal*, **336**, 491–5.

Deakin, T.A., Cade, J.E., Williams, R. and Greenwood, D.C. (2006) Structured patient education: the Diabetes X-PERT Programme makes a difference. *Diabetic Medicine*, **23**, 944–54.

DeFronzo, R.A., Ratner, R.E., Han, J., Kim, D.D., Fineman, M.S. and Baron, A.D. (2005) Effects of exenatide (exendin-4) on glycaemic control and weigh over 30 weeks in metformin-treated patients with type 2 diabetes. *Diabetes Care*, **28**, 1092–2000.

Department of Health (2001) *National Service Framework for Diabetes: Standards.* Department of Health, London.

Department of Health (2003) *National Service Framework for Diabetes: Delivery Strategy.* Department of Health, London.

Department of Health (2006a) Forecasting obesity to 2010. http://www.dh.gov.uk/en/ Publicationsandstatistics/Publications/PublicationsStatistics/DH_4138630 (accessed 21 January 2008).

Department of Health (2006b) http://www.dh.gov.uk/en/Publicationsandstatistics/ Publications/PublicationsPolicyAndGuidance/DH_4139673 (accessed 29 April 2008).

Department of Health (2007) Obesity general information. http://www.dh.gov.uk/en/Policyandguidance/Healthandsocialcaretopics/Obesity (accessed 22 January 2008).

Deville-Almond, J. (2003) An innovative approach to weight management. *Obesity in Practice*, **5**, 6–8.

Diabetes Control and Complications Trial Research Group (1993) The effect of intensive treatment of diabetes on the development and progression of long-term complications in insulin-dependent diabetes mellitus. *New England Journal of Medicine*, **326**, 683–9.

Diabetes Control and Complications Trial Research Group (1995) Effect of intensive therapy on the development and progression of diabetic nephropathy in the Diabetes Control and Complications Trial. *Kidney International*, **47**, 1703–20.

Diabetes Control and Complications Trial Research Group (1997) Hypoglycaemia in the Diabetes Control and Complications Trial. *Diabetes*, **46**, 271–86.

Diabetes UK (2001) Guidelines for the management of diabetic ketoacidosis in children and adolescents. http://www.diabetes.org.uk (accessed 22 July 2008).

Diabetes UK (2005) Type 2 diabetes and obesity: a heavy burden. Avaiable from: http:// www.diabetes.org.uk/Site_Search/?p=1andpr=114andandt1=obesityandt2=andt3=

andt4=andd1=andd2=andd3=andd4=andd5=andd6=andchk=00000100000 (accessed 23 November 2007).

Diabetes UK (2006a) Reports and statistics. http://www.diabetes.org.uk/Professionals/ Information_resources/Reports/Diabetes_prevalence_2006/ (accessed 21 June 2007).

Diabetes UK (2006b) Analogue insulin. http://www.diabetes.org/Guide-to-diabetes/ Guide_to_Diabetes_Archived_pages/Anal (accessed 6 July 2007).

Diabetes UK (2008) Year of care. http://www.diabetes.org.uk/Professionals/Year-of-Care/ (accessed 28 October 2008)

DIAMOND Project Group (2006) Incidence and trends of childhood Type 1 diabetes worldwide 1990–1999. *Diabetic Medicine*, **23**, 857–66.

Dinneen, S.F. (2008) Structured education for people with type 2 diabetes. *British Medical Journal*, **336**, 459–60.

Disability Discrimination Act (1995). http://www.opsi.gov.uk/acts/acts1995/1995050.htm (accessed 25 July 2007).

Dixon, J.B., Bhathal, P.S., Hughes, N.R. and O'Brien, P.E. (2004) Nonalcoholic fatty liver disease: improvement in liver histological analysis with weight loss. *Hepatology*, **39**, 1647–54.

Donnelly, R. (2005) Managing cardiovascular risk in patients with diabetes. *The British Journal of Diabetes and Vascular Disease*, **5**, 325–9.

Drucker, D.J. (2007) The role of gut hormones in glucose homeostasis. *Journal of Clinical Investigation*, **117**, 24–32.

Drucker, D.J . and Nauck, M.A. (2006) The incretin system: glucagon-like peptide-1 receptor agonists and dipeptidyl peptidase-4 inhibitors in type 2 diabetes. *The Lancet*, **368**, 1696–705.

Edmonds, M.E. and Foster, A.V.M. (2000) *Managing the Diabetic Foot*. Blackwell Science, Oxford.

Elliott, R.B., Reddy, S.N., Bibby, N.J. and Kida, K. (1988) Dietary prevention of diabetes in the non-obese diabetic mouse. *Diabetologia*, **31**, 62–4.

Erdmann, E. (2007) Statin plus thiazolidinedione use in patients with diabetes at high cardiovascular risk. *The British Journal of Diabetes and Vascular Disease*, **7**, 211–16.

EURODIAB Substudy 2 Study Group (1999) Vitamin D supplement in early childhood and risk for Type 1 (insulin-dependent) diabetes mellitus. *Diabetologia*, **42**, 51–4.

European Association for the Study of the Liver (2000a) EASL International Consensus Conference of Haemochromatosis – Part III. Jury document. *Journal of Hepatology*, **33**, 496–504.

European Association for the Study of the Liver (2000b) EASL International Consensus Conference of Haemochromatosis – Part II. Expert document. *Journal of Hepatology*, **33**, 487–96.

Evans, J.J., Youngren, J.F. and Goldfine, I.D. (2004) Effective treatments for insulin resistance: trim the fat and douse the fire. *Trends in Endocrinology and Metabolism*, **15**, 425–31.

Faideau, B., Larger, E., Lepault, F., Carel, J.C. and Boitard, C. (2005) Role of β-cells in Type 1 diabetes pathogenesis. *Diabetes*, **54**, S87–96.

Fanelli, C., Pampanelli, S., Epifano, L., *et al.* (1994) Relative roles of insulin and hypoglycaemia on induction of neuroendocrine responses to, symptoms of, and deterioration of cognitive function in hypoglycaemia in male and female humans. *Diabetologia*, **37**, 797–807.

Feder, J.N., Gnirke, A., Thomas, W., *et al.* (1996) A novel MHC class 1-like gene is mutated in patients with hereditary haemochromatosis. *Nature Genetics*, **13**, 399–408.

Fioretto, P., Bruseghin, M., Barzon, I., Arboit, M. and Dalla Vestra, M. (2007) Diabetic nephropathy: an update on renal structure. *International Congress Series*, **1303**, 51–9.

Foresight (2007) Tackling obesities: future choices. http://www.foresight.gov.ukproject (accessed 21 January 2008).

Foreyt, J.P. and Poston, C. (1999) The challenge of diet, exercise and lifestyle modification in the management of the obese diabetic patient. *International Journal of Obesity*, **7**, S5–11.

Foster H (2004) *Easy GI Diet*. Hamlyn, London.

Fraser, D.J. and Phillips, A.O. (2007) Diabetic nephropathy. *Medicine*, **35**, 503–6.

French, G. (2000) Clinical management of diabetes mellitus during anaesthesia and surgery. *Practical Procedures*, **11**, 1–3.

Galbraith, A., Bullock, S., Manias, E., Hunt, B. and Richards A (1999) *Fundamentals of Pharmacology*. Addison Wesley Longman, Harlow.

Gallop, R. and Renton, H. (2005) *The GI Guide*. Virgin Books, London.

Hales, C.N. and Barker, D.J.P. (2001) The thrifty phenotype hypothesis. *British Medical Bulletin*, **60**, 5–20.

Gillespie, G.L. and Campbell, M. (2002) Diabetic ketoacidosis: rapid identification, treatment, and education can improve survival rates. *American Journal of Nursing*, **102**, 13–16.

Gillespie, K.M., Bain, S.C., Barnett, A.H., Bingley, P.J., Christie, M.R. and Gill, G.V. (2004) The rising incidence of childhood type 1 diabetes and reduction contribution of high-risk HLA haplotypes. *The Lancet*, **364**, 1699–700.

Goldman, L. (1995) Cardiac risk in non cardiac surgery: an update. *Anaesthesia and Analgesia*, **80**, 810–20.

Goldrick, B.A. (2003) Surgical-site infections. *American Journal of Nursing*, **103**, 64A.

Greenstein, A., Tavaloli, M., Mojaddidi, M., Al-Sunni, A., Matfin, G. and Malik, R.A. (2007) Microvascular complications: evaluation and monitoring relevance to clinical practice, clinical trials, and drug development. *The British Journal of Diabetes and Vascular Disease*, **7**, 166–71.

Gross, E.R., LaDisa, J.F., Weihrauch, D., *et al.* (2003) Reactive oxygen species modulate coronary wall shear stress and endothelial function during hyperglycaemia. *American Journal of Physiology*, **284**, H1552–9.

Gross, J.L., Canani, L.H., de Azevedo, M.J., Caramori, M.L., Silveiro, S.P. and Zelmanovitz, T. (2005) Diabetic nephropathy: diagnosis, prevention and treatment. *Diabetes Care*, **28**, 164–76.

Grundy, S.M., Cleeman, J.I., Donato, K.A., *et al.* (2005) Diagnosis and management of the metabolic syndrome. *Circulation*, **112**, 2735–52.

Guenaga, K., Atallah, A.N., Castro, A.A., Matos, D.D.M. and Wille-Jørgensen, P. (2007) Mechanical bowel preparation for elective colorectal surgery. *Cochrane Database of Systematic Reviews*, Issue 4. The Cochrane Collaboration, John Wiley, London.

Guidorizzi de Siqueira, A.C., Cotrim, H.P., Rocha, R., *et al.* (2005) Non-alcoholic fatty liver disease and insulin resistance: importance of risk factors and histological spectrum. *European Journal of Gastroenterology and Hepatology*, 17, 837–41.

Haag, B.L. (2000) Presurgical management of the patient with diabetes. In: *Medical Management of Diabetes* (eds J.L. Leahy, N.G. Clark and W.T. Cefalu), pp. 631–9. Marcel Dekker, New York.

Haemochromatosis Society (2006) Haemochromatosis. An iron overload disorder. http://www.ghsoc.org/pates/print.html (accessed 2 May 2008).

Haffner, S.M., Lehto, S., Ronnemaa, T., Pyorala, K. and Laakso, M. (1998) Mortality from coronary heart disease in subjects with type 2 diabetes and in nondiabetic subjects with and without prior myocardial infarction. *New England Journal of Medicine*, 339, 229–34.

Hand, H. (2000) The development of diabetic ketoacidosis. *Nursing Standard*, 15, 47–55.

Happich, M., Landfraf, R., Piehlmeier, W., Falkenstein, P. and Stamentis, S. (2008) The economic burden of nephropathy in diabetic patients in Germany 2002. *Diabetes Research and Clinical Practice*, 80, 34–9.

Haslam, D.W. and James, W.P.T. (2005) Obesity. *The Lancet*, 366, 1197–209.

Heart Protection Study Collaborative Group (2002) MRC/BHF Heart Protection Study of cholesterol lowering with simvastatin in 20,536 high-risk individuals: a randomised placebo-controlled trial. *The Lancet*, 360, 7–22.

Henriksen, O.M., Prahl, J.B., Røder, M.E. and Svendsen, O.L. (2006) Treatment of diabetic ketoacidosis in adults in Denmark: a national survey. *Diabetes Research and Clinical Practice*, 77, 113–19.

Hermann, R., Knip, M., Veijola, R., *et al.* (2003) Temporal changes in the frequencies of HLA genotypes in patients with type 1 diabetes – indication of an increased environmental pressure? *Diabetologia*, 46, 420–25.

Herrero, J.I., Quiroga, J., Sangro, B., *et al.* (2003) Conversion from calcineurin inhibitors to mycophenolate mofetil in liver transplant recipients with diabetes mellitus. *Transplantation Proceedings*, 35, 1877–99.

Hettiarachchi, K.D., Zimmet, P.Z. and Myers, M.A. (2004) Transplacental exposure to bafilomycin disrupts pancreatic islet organogenesis and accelerates diabetes onset in NOD mice. *Journal of Autoimmunity*, 22, 287–96.

Hickman, I.J., Russell, A.J., Prins, J.B. and Macdonald, G.A. (2008) Should patients with type 2 diabetes and raised liver enzymes be referred for further evaluation of liver disease? *Diabetes Research and Clinical Practice*, 80, e10–e12.

Hill, A. (2002) Continuous intravenous insulin infusion in patients with diabetes after cardiac surgery. *Clinical Nurse Specialist*, 16, 93–5.

Hirose, A., Ono, M., Saibara, T., *et al.* (2007) Angiotensin II type 1 receptor blocker inhibits fibrosis in rat nonalcoholic steatohepatitis. *Hepatology*, 45, 1375–81.

Hoek, J.B. and Pastorino, J.G. (2002) Ethanol, oxidative stress, and cytokine-induced liver cell injury. *Alcohol*, 27, 63–9.

Hovind, P., Tarnow, L., Rossing, P., Jensen, B.R., Graae, M., Torp, I., *et al.* (2004) Predictors of the development of microalbuminuria and macroalbuminuria in patients with type 1 diabetes: inception cohort study. *British Medical Journal*, **328**, 1105–8.

Humphries, C. (2002) *The Hugely Better Calorie Counter Essentials.* Foulsham, Berkshire.

IDF (2005) The International Diabetes Federation (IDF) consensus worldwide definition of the metabolic syndrome. April 14, 2005. http://www.idf.org/webdata/docs/Metac_syndrome_def.pdf (accessed 22 January 2008).

IDF (2007) The International Diabetes Federation (IDF) recommends tighter control of blood glucose levels after meals in people with diabetes. Press release. http://www.idf.org/home/index.cfm?unode=BE8B67AD-1C8B-405C-A327-CB0B40272 (accessed 28 November 2007).

Ihnat, M.A., Thorpe, J.E. and Ceriello, A. (2007) Hypothesis: the 'metabolic memory', the new challenge of diabetes. *Diabetic Medicine*, **24**, 582–6.

Ilag, L.L., Kronick, S., Ernst, R.D., *et al.* (2003) Impact of a critical pathway on inpatient management of diabetic ketoacidosis. *Diabetes Research and Clinical Practice*, **62**, 1, 23–32.

JBS (2005) Joint British Societies' guidelines on prevention of cardiovascular disease in clinical practice. *Heart*, **91**, (Suppl. 5), v1–v52.

Jellish, W.S., Kartha, V., Fluder, E. and Slogoff, S. (2005) Effects of metoclopramide on gastric fluid volumes in diabetic patients who have fasted before elective surgery. *Anaesthesiology*, **102**, 904–9.

Jerreat, L. (2003) *Diabetes for Nurses.* John Wiley, London.

Jones, D.B. and Crosby, I. (1996) Proliferative lymphocyte responses to virus antigens homologous to GAD65 in IDDM. *Diabetologia*, **39**,1318–24.

Kaila, B., Dean, H.J., Schroeder, M. and Taback, S.P. (2003) HLA, day care attendance and socio-economic status in young patients with type 1 diabetes. *Diabetic Medicine*, **20**, 777–80.

Karci, A., Tasdogen, A., Erkin, Y., Akta, G. and Elar, Z. (2004) The analgesic effect of morphine on postoperative pain in diabetic patients. *Acta Anaesthesiologica Scandinavica*, **48**, 619–24.

Katzung, B.G. (1998) *Basic and Clinical Pharmacology*, 7th edn. Appleton and Lange, Connecticut.

Kershaw, E.E. and Flier, J.S. (2004) Adipose tissue as an endocrine organ. *Journal of Clinical Endocrinology Metabolism*, **84**, 2548–56.

Kersten, J.R., Warltier, D.C. and Pagel, P.S. (2005) Aggressive control of intraoperative blood glucose concentration; editorial view. *Anaesthesiology*, **103**, 677–8.

Kettyle, W.M. and Arky, R.A. (1998) *Endocrine Pathophysiology.* Lippincott–Raven, New York.

Khaodhiar, L., Dinh, T., Schomacker, K., *et al.* (2007) The use of medical hyperspectral technology to evaluate microcirculatory changes in diabetic foot ulcers and to predict clinical outcomes. *Diabetes Care*, **30**, 903–10.

Kirby, M.G. (2006) NICE and hypertension – the judge's decision is final! *The British Journal of Diabetes and Vascular Disease*, **6**, 177–9.

Kitabchi, A.E. and Wall, B.M. (1999) Management of diabetic ketoacidosis. *American Family Physician*, **60**, 455–64.

Knowler, W.C., Barrett-Connor, E., Fowler, S.E., *et al.* (2002) Reduction of the incidence of type 2 diabetes with lifestyle intervention or metformin. *New England Journal of Medicine*, **346**, 393–403.

Kumar, R. and Winocour, P.H. (2005) Dual blockade of the renin angiotensin system in diabetes – rationale and risks. *The British Journal of Diabetes and Vascular Disease*, **5**, 266–71.

Kravitz, S.R., McGuire, J.B. and Sharma, S. (2007) The treatment of diabetic foot ulcers: reviewing the literature and a surgical algorithm. *Skin and Wound*, **20**, 227–37.

Levetan, C.S., Passaro, M.D., Jablonski, K.A. and Ratner, R.E. (1999) Effect of physician speciality on outcomes in DKA. *Diabetes Care*, **22**, 1790–5.

Levin, A., Thompson, C., Ethier, J., *et al.* (1999) Left ventricular mass index increase in early renal disease: impact of decline in haemoglobin. *American Journal of Kidney Diseases*, **34**, 125–34.

Levy, D. (2006) *Practical Diabetes*, 2nd edn. Altman, Hertfordshire.

Li, Z., Yang, S., Lin, H., *et al.* (2003) Probiotics and antibodies to TNF inhibit inflammatory activity and improve NAFLD. *Hepatology*, **37**, 343–50.

Lieber, C.S., Leo, M.A., Mak, K.M., *et al.* (2004) Model of nonalcoholic steatohepatitis. *American Journal of Clinical Nutrition*, **79**, 502–9.

Lilly, L.S. (2006) *Pathophysiology of Heart Disease. A Collaborative Project of Medical Students and Faculty* (4th edn). Lippincott Williams and Wilkins, London.

Lunt, H. and Brown, J.L.J. (1996) Self-reported changes in capillary glucose and insulin requirements during the menstrual cycle. *Diabetic Medicine*, **13**, 525–30.

Maggio, C.A. and Pi-Sunyer, F.X. (1997) The prevention and treatment of obesity. Application to type 2 diabetes. *Diabetes Care*, **20**, 1744–66.

Malmberg, K.A., Ryden, L., Efendic, S., *et al.* on behalf of the DIGAMI Study Group (1997) Prospective randomised study of intensive insulin treatment on long term survival after acute myocardial infraction in patients with diabetes. *British Medical Journal*, **314**, 1512–15.

Malmberg, K.A., Ryden, L., Wedel, H., *et al.* for the DIGAMI 2 Investigators (2005) Intense metabolic control by means of insulin in patients with diabetes mellitus and acute myocardial infarction (DIGAMI 2): effects on morbidity and mortality. *European Heart Journal*, **26**, 650–61.

Marchetti, P. (2005) New-onset diabetes after liver transplantation: from pathogenesis to management. *Liver Transplantation*, **11**, 612–20.

Marieb, E.N. (2001) *Human Anatomy and Physiology*, 5th edn. Addison Wesley Longman, London.

Marks, J.B. (2003) Perioperative management of diabetes. *American Family Physician*, **67**, 93–100.

Marshall, S.M. and Flyvbjerg, A. (2006) Prevention and early detection of vascular complications of diabetes. *British Medical Journal*, **333**, 475–80.

Martini, F. (2006) *Fundamentals of Anatomy and Physiology*, 7th edn. Benjamin-Cummings, San Francisco.

Martini, F.H. and Karleskint, G. (1998) *Foundations of Anatomy and Physiology*. Prentice Hall, Upper Saddle River, NJ.

Matfin, G. (2007) Challenges in developing therapies for the metabolic syndrome. *The British Journal of Diabetes and Vascular Disease*, 7, 152–6.

McAvoy, N., Ferguson, J.W., Campbell, I.W. and Hayes, P.C. (2006) Non-alcoholic fatty liver disease: natural history, pathogenesis and treatment. *The British Journal of Diabetes and Vascular Disease*, 6, 251–60.

McClain, D.A., Abraham, D., Rogers, J., *et al.* (2006) High prevalence of abnormal glucose homeostasis secondary to decreased insulin secretion in individuals with hereditary haemochromatosis. *Diabetologia*, **49**, 1661–9.

McCoubrey, A.S. (2007) The use of mechanical bowel preparation in elective colorectal surgery. *Ulster Medical Journal*, **76**, 127–30.

McNeely, M.J., Boyko, E.J., Ahroni, J.H., Reiber, G., Smith, D.G. and Pecoraro, R.E. (1995) The independent contributions of diabetic neuropathy and vasculopathy in foot ulceration: how great are the risks? *Diabetes Care*, **18**, 216–19.

Mende, C. (2006) Improving antihypertensive therapy in patients with diabetic nephropathy. *Southern Medical Journal*, **99**, 150–7.

Menser, M.A., Forrest, J.M. and Bransby, R.D. (1978) Rubella infection and diabetes mellitus. *The Lancet*, **1**, 57–60.

Mitrakou, A., Ryan, C., Veneman, T., *et al.* (1991) Hierarchy of glycemic thresholds for counterregulatory hormone secretion, symptoms and cerebral dysfunction. *American Journal of Physiology Endocrinology and Metabolism*, **260**, E67–E74.

Mogensen, C.E. (2003) Microalbuminuria and hypertension with a focus on type 1 and type 2 diabetes. *Journal of International Medicine*, **254**, 45–66.

Mokdad, A.H., Ford, E.S. and Bowman, B.A. (2000) Diabetes trends in the U.S 1990–1998. *Diabetes Care*, **23**, 1278–83.

Montgomery, M.P., Kamel, F., Saldana, T.M., Alvanja, M.C.R. and Sandler, D.P. (2008) Incident diabetes and pesticide exposure among licensed pesticide applicators: agricultural health study, 1993–2003. *American Journal of Epidemiology*, **67**, 1235–46.

Mosby's (2002) *Medical, Nursing and Allied Health Dictionary*, 6th edn. Mosby, London.

Najarian, J., Swavely, D., Wilson, E. *et al.* (2005) Improving outcomes for diabetic patients undergoing vascular surgery. *Diabetes Spectrum*, **18**, 53–60.

Nakamura, T., Ushiyama, C., Suzuki, S., *et al.* (2000) Urinary excretion of podocytes in patients with diabetic nephropathy. *Nephrology Dialysis Transplantation*, **15**, 1379–83.

Nathan, D.M., Buse, J.B., Davidson, M.B., *et al.* (2006) Management of hyperglycaemia in type 2 diabetes: a consensus algorithm for the initiation and adjustment of therapy. A consensus statement from the American Diabetes Association and the European Association for the Study of Diabetes. *Diabetologia*, **49**, 1711–21.

National Diabetes Support Team (2008) Partners in care: a guide to implementing a care planning approach to diabetes care. National Diabetes Support Team, reference NDST062. http://www.diabetes.nhs.uk/news-1/Partners%20in%20Care.pdf (accessed 29 October 2008).

National Heart Lung and Blood Institute (1998) Clinical guidelines on the identification, evaluation and treatment of overweight and obesity in adults. The Evidence Report. National Institutes of Health, Bethesda, Maryland.

National Kidney Foundation (2004) K/DOQI clinical practice guidelines on hypertension and antihypertensive agents in chronic kidney disease. *American Journal of Kidney Disease*, **43** (Suppl. 1), S1–290.

Neligan, P.J. and Fleisher. L.A. (2006) Obesity and diabetes. Evidence of increased perioperative risk? *Anaesthesiology*, **104**, 398–9.

NICE (2003) Guidance on the use of patient-education models for diabetes. Technology Appraisal Guidance 60. National Institute for Health and Clinical Excellence, London. http://www.nice.org.uk/nicemedia (accessed 2 July 2008).

NICE (2006) Inhaled insulin for the treatment of diabetes (types 1 and 2). Technology Appraisal Guidance 113. National Institute for Health and Clinical Excellence, London.

NICE (2008) Type 2 diabetes. The management of type 2 diabetes. Clinical Guideline 66. National Institute for Health and Clinical Excellence, London. http://www.nice.org.uk/guidance/index.jsp?action=downloadando=40754 (accessed 13 October 2008).

Nissen, S.E. and Wolski, K. (2007) Effect of Rosiglitazone on risk of myocardial infarction and death from cardiovascular disease. *The New England Journal of Medicine*, **356**, 2457–71.

Norris, J.M. and Scott, F.W. (1996) A meta-analysis of infant diet and insulin-dependent diabetes mellitus: do biases play a role? *Epidemiology*, **7**, 87–92.

Norris, S.L., Engelgau, M.M. and Venkat Narayan, K.M. (2001) Review: self management training in type 2 diabetes mellitus is effective in the short term. *American College of Physicians Journal Club*, Sept/Oct, p. 45.

Norris, S.L., Lau, J., Smith, S.J., Schmid, C.H. and Engelgau, M.M. (2002) Self-management education for adults with type 2 diabetes: a meta-analysis of the effect on glycaemic control. *Diabetes Care*, **25**, 1159–71.

Norris, S., Zhang, X., Avenell, A., *et al.* (2004) Long-term effectiveness of lifestyle and behavioural weight loss interventions in adults with type 2 diabetes: a meta-analysis. *The American Journal of Medicine*, **117**, 762–74.

Nutrition Subcommittee of the Diabetes Care Advisory Committee of Diabetes UK (2003) The implementation of nutritional advice for people with diabetes. *Diabetic Medicine*, **20**, 786–807.

Olveira-Fuster, G., Olvera-Marquez, P., Carral-Sanlaureano, F., Gonzalez-Romero. S., Aguilar-Diosdado. M. and Soriguer-Escofet, F. (2004) Excess hospitalizations, hospital days, and inpatient costs among people with diabetes in Andalusia, Spain. *Diabetes Care*, **27**, 1904–9.

Ouattara, A., Lecomte, P., Le Manach, Y., *et al.* (2005) Poor intraoperative blood glucose control is associated with a worsened hospital outcome after cardiac surgery in diabetic patients. *Anaesthesiology*, **103**, 687–94.

Page, S.R. and Hall, G.M. (1999) *Diabetes Emergency and Hospital Management*. BMJ Books, London.

Picardi, A., D'Avola, D., Gentilucci, U.V., *et al.* (2006) Diabetes in chronic liver disease: from old concepts to new evidence. *Diabetes Metabolism Research and Reviews*, **22**, 274–83.

Pittas, A.G., Siegel, R.D. and Lau, J. (2004) Insulin therapy for critically ill hospitalized patients. A meta-analysis of randomised controlled trials. *Archives of Internal Medicine*, **164**, 2005–11.

Plodkowski, R.A. and Edelman, S.V. (2001) Pre-surgical evaluation of diabetic patients. *Clinical Diabetes*, **19**, 92–5.

Pozzilli, P. and Mario, U.D. (2001) Autoimmune diabetes not requiring insulin at diagnosis (Latent Autoimmune Diabetes of the Adult). *Diabetes Care*, **24**, 1460–7.

Quality Outcomes Framework (2006/07) The Quality Outcomes Framework. http://www.ic.nhs.uk/our-services/improving-patient-care/the-quality-and-outcomes-framework-qof-2006–07 (accessed 15 July 2008).

Reichstein, L., Labrenz, S., Ziegler, D. and Martin, S. (2005) Effective treatment of symptomatic diabetic polyneuropathy by high-frequency external muscle stimulation. *Diabetologia*, **48**, 824–8.

Reilly, J.J. (2004) Prevention of obesity in children. *Obesity in Practice*, **6**, 6–8.

Rennke, H.G. and Denker, B.M. (2007) *Renal Pathophysiology: The Essentials*, 2nd edn. Lippincott, Williams and Wilkins, London.

Richardson, T., Weiss, M., Thomas, P. and Kerr, D. (2005) Day after the night before. *Diabetes Care*, **28**, 1801–2.

Rimm, E.B., Chan, J., Stampter, M.J., Colditz, G.A. and Willett, W.C. (1995) Prospective study of cigarette smoking, alcohol use, and the risk of diabetes in men. *British Medical Journal*, **310**, 555–9.

Rincon, J., Krook, A., Galuska, D., Walberg-Henriksson, H. and Sierath, J.R. (1999) Altered skeletal muscle glucose transport and blood lipids in habitual cigarette smokers. *Clinical Physiology*, **19**, 135–42.

Rodacki, M., Pereira, J.R.D., de Oliveira, A.M.N., *et al.* (2007) Ethnicity and young age influence the frequency of diabetic ketoacidosis at the onset of type 1 diabetes. *Diabetes Research and Clinical Practice*, **78**, 259–62.

Rorsman, P. (2005) Insulin secretion: function and therapy of pancreatic beta-cells in diabetes. *The British Journal of Diabetes and Vascular Disease*, **5**, 187–91.

Sampson, M.J., Crowle, T., Dhatariaya, K., *et al.* (2006) Trends in bed occupancy for inpatients with diabetes before and after the introduction of a diabetes inpatient specialist nurse service. *Diabetic Medicine*, **23**, 1008–15.

Sato, T., Inagaki, A., Uchida, K., *et al.* (2003) Diabetes mellitus after transplant: relationship to pretransplant glucose metabolism and tacrolimus or cyclosporine A based therapy. *Transplantation*, **76**, 1320–6.

Savage, M.W. and Kilvert, A. (2006) ABCD guidelines for the management of hyperglycaemic emergencies in adults. *Practical Diabetes International*, **23**, 227–31.

Sawaki, H., Terasaki, J., Fujita, A., *et al.* (2008) A renoprotective effect of low dose losartan in patients with type 2 diabetes. *Diabetes Research and Clinical Practice*, **79**, 86–90.

Schwarze, C.P. and Dunger, D.B. (2005) Management of early diabetic nephropathy in adolescents with type 1 diabetes mellitus. *Practical Diabetes International*, **22**, 65–9.

Sharma, A., Kumar, S., Sharma, N., Jain, S. and Varma, S. (2007) Bilateral parietal lobe hemorrhage in a patient with diabetic ketoacidosis. *Diabetes Research and Clinical Practice*, **75**, 379–80.

Shepherd, P.R. and Kahn, B.B. (1999) Glucose transporters and insulin action. *New England Journal of Medicine*, **341**, 248–57.

Smithies, O. (2003) Why the kidney glomerulus does not clog: a gel permeation/diffusion hypothesis of renal function. *The Proceedings of the National Academy of Sciences Online USA*, **100**, 4180–213.

Song, S.H. and Hardisty, C.A. (2007) Cardiovascular risk profile of early and later onset type 2 diabetes. *Practical Diabetes International*, **24**, 20–4.

Soule, J.L., Olyaei, A.J., Boslaugh, T., *et al.* (2005) Hepatitis C infection increases the risk of new-onset diabetes after transplantation in liver allograft recipients. *American Journal of Surgery*, **189**, 552–7.

Stehouwer, C.D.A., Nauta, J.J.P., Zeldenrust, G.C., *et al.* (1992) Urinary albumin excretion, cardiovascular disease, and endothelial dysfunction in non-insulin-dependent diabetes mellitus. *The Lancet*, **340**, 319–23.

Stene, L.C., Ulriksen, J., Magnus, P. and Joner, G. (2000) Use of cod liver oil during pregnancy associated with lower risk of Type 1 diabetes in the offspring. *Diabetologia*, **43**, 1093–8.

Stratton, I.M., Adler, A.I., Neil, H.A.W., *et al.* on behalf of the UK Prospective Diabetes Study Centre (2000) Association of glycaemia with macrovascular and microvascular complications of type 2 diabetes (UKPDS 35): prospective observational study. *British Medical Journal*, **321**, 405–12.

Tamas, G., Tabak, A.G., Vargha, P. and Kerenyi, Z. (1996) Effect of menstrual cycle on insulin demand in IDDM women. *Diabetologia*, **39** (Suppl. 1):A52 (Abstract 188).

Targher, G., Bertolini, L., Poli, F., *et al.* (2005) Nonalcoholic fatty liver disease and risk of future cardiovascular events among type 2 diabetic patients. *Diabetes*, **54**, 3541–6.

Tavill, A.S. (2001) Diagnosis and management of haemochromatosis. *Hepatology*, **33**, 1321–8.

Tesfaye, S. and Kempler, P. (2005) Painful diabetic neuropathy. *Diabetologia*, **48**, 805–7.

The Diabetes Information Jigsaw (2006) http://www.abpi.org.uk/%2Fpublications%2Fpdfs%2Fdiabetes_jigsaw.pdf (accessed 6 June 2008).

Thomson, F.J., Masson, E.A., Leeming, J.T. and Boulton, A.J.M. (1991) Lack of knowledge of symptoms of hypoglycaemia by elderly diabetic patients. *Age and Ageing*, **20**, 404–6.

Toeller, M., Buyken, A., Heitkamp, G., *et al.* and the EURODIAB IDDM Complications Study Group (1997) Protein intake and urinary excretion rates in the EURODIAB IDDM Complications Study. *Diabetologia*, **40**, 1219–26.

UK Prospective Diabetes Study (1998) Tight blood pressure control and risk of macrovascular and microvascular complications in type 2 diabetes (UKPDS 38). *British Medical Journal*; **317**, 703–13.

Umpierrez, G.E., Cuervo, R., Karabell, A., Latif, K., Freire, A.X. and Kitabchi, A.E. (2004) Treatment of diabetic ketoacidosis with subcutaneous insulin aspart. *Diabetes Care*, **27**, 1873–8.

Vaarala, O., Knip, M., Paronen, J., *et al.* (1999) Cow's milk formula feeding induces primary immunization to insulin in infants at genetic risk for type 1 diabetes. *Diabetes*, **48**, 1389–94.

Valerkou, S. (2006) Structured education for people with type 1 diabetes. *Diabetes Update*, Winter, 38–40.

Van den Berghe, G. (2005) Insulin vs. strict blood glucose control to achieve a survival benefit after AMI? *European Heart Journal*, **26**, 639–41.

Van den Berghe, G., Wouters, P., Weekers, F., *et al.* (2001) Intensive insulin therapy in critically ill patients. *New England Journal of Medicine*, **345**, 1359–67.

Van de Wiel, A. (2004) Diabetes mellitus and alcohol. *Diabetes Metabolism Research and Reviews*, **20**, 263–7.

Vora, J. and Weston, C. (2006) BENEDICT: primary prevention of microalbuminuria in hypertensive type 2 diabetics. *The British Journal of Diabetes and Vascular Disease*, **6**, 84–6.

Wadden, T.A., Berkowitz, R.I., Womble, L.G., *et al.* (2005) Randomised trial of lifestyle modification and pharmacotherapy for obesity. *New England Journal of Medicine*, **353**, 2111–20.

Walker, E.F. (1999) Management of diabetes and hyperglycaemia during myocardial infarction: review of the literature. *Intensive and Critical Care Nursing*, **15**, 259–65.

Wallace, T.M., Meston, N.M., Gardner, S.G. and Matthews, D.R. (2001) The hospital and home use of a 30 second hand-held blood ketone meter: guidelines for clinical practice. *Diabetic Medicine*, **18**, 640–45.

Wang, C.S., Wang, S.T., Yao, W.J., Chang, T.T. and Chou, P. (2007) Hepatitis C virus infection and the development of type 2 diabetes in a community-based longitudinal study. *American Journal of Epidemiology*, **166**, 196–203.

WHO (1980) WHO Expert Committee on Diabetes Mellitus. Second Report. Technical Report Series 646. World Health Organization, Geneva.

WHO (1999) Definition, diagnosis and classification of diabetes mellitus and its complications. World Health Organization, Geneva. http://www.who.int/diabetes/publications/Definition%20and%20diagnosis%20of%20diabetes_new.pdf (accessed 15 March 2007).

WHO (2006) Definition and diagnosis of diabetes mellitus and intermediate hyperglycaemia: report of a WHO/IDF consultation. World Health Organization/International Diabetes Federation. http://www.who.int/diabetes/publications (accessed 5 May 2008).

Wiernsperger, N.F. (2007) 50 years later: is metformin a vascular drug with antidiabetic properties? *The British Journal of Diabetes and Vascular Disease*, **7**, 204–10.

Wikipedia (2007) Insulin analog. http://en.wikipedia.org/wik/insulin_analog (accessed 30 June 2007).

Wild, S., Roglic, G., Green, A., Sicree, R. and King, H. (2004) Global prevalence of diabetes: estimates of the year 2000 and projections for 2030. *Diabetes Care*, **27**, 1047–53.

Will, J.C., Galuska, A., Ford, E.S., Mokdad, A., Calle, E.E. (2001) Cigarette smoking and diabetes mellitus: evidence of a positive association from a large prospective cohort study. *International Journal of Epidemiology*, **30**, 540–6.

Williams, B., Poulter, N.R. and Brown, M.J. (2004) Guidelines for management of hypertension: report of the fourth working party of the British Hypertensive Society. *Journal of Human Hypertension*, **18**, 139–85.

Williams, G. and Pickup, J.C. (2004) *Handbook of Diabetes*, 3rd edn. Blackwell Publishing, Oxford.

Woerle, H.J., Neumann, C., Zschau, S., *et al.* (2006) Impact of fasting and postprandial glycemia on overall glycemic control in type 2 diabetes. Importance of postprandial glycemia to achieve target HbA1c levels. *Diabetes Research and Clinical Practice*, **77**, 280–5.

Wolf, G., Chen, S. and Ziyadeh, F.N. (2005) From the periphery of the glomerular capillary wall to the centre of disease. *Diabetes*, **54**, 1626–34.

Yunianingtias, D. and Volker, D. (2006) Nutritional aspects of non-alcoholic steatohepatitis treatment. *Nutrition and Dietetics*, **63**, 79–90.

Zammitt, N.N. and Frier, B.M. (2005) Hypoglycaemia in Type 2 diabetes. *Diabetes Care*, **28**, 2948–61.

Zimmet, P.Z., Tuomi, T., Mackay, R., *et al.* (1994) Latent autoimmune diabetes mellitus in adults (LADA): the role of antibodies to glutamic acid decarboxylase in diagnosis and prediction of insulin dependency. *Diabetic Medicine*, **11**, 299–303.

Index

Numbers in *italic* refer to pages where the topic is found only in the figure. Numbers in **bold** refer to pages where the topic is to be found only in the table.